Child of Mine:

Caring for the Skin and Hair of Your Adopted Child

By Brooke Jackson, M.D.

Windy City Publishers
2118 Plum Grove Rd., #349
Rolling Meadows, IL 60008
www.windycitypublishers.com

Published in the United States of America

10 9 8 7 6 5 4 3 2 1

First Edition: 2012

Library of Congress Control Number: 2012931198

ISBN: 978-1-935766-51-3

Cover Production by Amanda Inkinen
Cover Image by Larry Williams/Blend Images/Getty Images

Windy City Publishers
Chicago

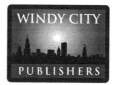

Dedication

This book is dedicated to family:
my always-supportive and loving husband, James,
and our three children, Reese, Avery, and Myles.

You fill my heart with unimaginable joy.

FOREWORD

This book is all about caring for the skin and hair of adopted children. It is a work of heart and art born from my personal experience as an adoptive mother of three (twin girls and a boy) and my professional experience as a board-certified dermatologist (a physician who specializes in treating disorders of the hair, skin, and nails).

As an adoptive mother of three, I am an adoption advocate. I also raise funds to support our adoption agency, which has placed more than 14,000 children since 1923. I ran my ninth marathon in 2010 (the Bank of America Chicago Marathon) to raise funds and create support for the Cradle Foundation and the Ardythe and Gale Sayers Center for African American Adoption, part of the Cradle. My husband and I volunteer as guest speakers for the Cradle, sharing our adoption story with prospective adoptive parents. Additionally, I lecture and teach workshops to newly adoptive parents about hair and skin care for adopted children.

Adopting a child brings great joy. Yet a child who doesn't share your medical history or background may have skin, scalp, and hair issues that are unfamiliar to you. Helpful birth-parent history and medical information may be limited or unavailable. In this guide to caring for the hair and skin of your adopted child, you'll learn about hair, scalp, and skin issues, with instructions for at-home solutions and how to know when you should seek the advice and care of a medical professional. When your child has a skin or hair concern, you'll be able to check the index and quickly get the solution or guidance that you need. You'll learn which products to use and which to avoid. Lastly, I'll share resources for hair and skin care that may not be available in your area.

Knowledge is power. Lovingly caring for and treating the skin and hair of your beautiful adopted child or children will be so much easier with the information in this book. It is my delight and privilege to share with you the knowledge you need to care for your adopted child's hair and skin.

TABLE OF CONTENTS

PART I: THE SKIN

About Skin...1

Skin Types 3

Skin FAQs 5

Getting Started—Basic Skin Care.................................... 9

Skin-Care Kit 14

Skin Issues from A to Z...15

Dry Skin (Xerosis Cutis)..16

Atopic Dermatitis (Eczema)..18

Keratosis Pilaris 22

Intertrigo/Diaper Rash 24

Acne: Neonatal and Infant.. 26

Infantile Acne 28

Acne.. 30

Seborrheic Dermatitis (Dandruff/Cradle Cap) 32

Skin Infection 34

Moles.. 35

Warts... 37

Molluscum Contagiosum 39

Birthmarks... 41

Café au Lait Spots... 45

Neurofibromatosis 47

Sun Damage... 49

Sunburn.. 53

Sun Protection Kit.. 55

Pediatric Skin Cancer 56

PART II: THE HAIR AND SCALP

About Hair 61

Hair Types 62

Hair FAQs 64

Getting Started: Basic Hair Care 70

Hair Care Kit 82

Hair Issues from A to Z 83

Cradle Cap—Seborrheic Dermatitis 84

Dandruff—Seborrhea 86

Tinea Capitis/Ringworm 88

Folliculitis 90

Head Lice/Pediculosis 92

Hair Loss 96

Hair Damage 98

Scalp Damage 101

Conclusion 103

Skin Resources 104

Hair Resources 106

Skin & Hair Glossary 107

Appendix 109

Index 110

Part 1: The Skin

About Skin

THE SKIN IS THE BODY'S LARGEST ORGAN—spanning approximately twenty square feet in an adult—with both structural and functional roles. Because our skin provides a barrier between our internal organs and the outside world, it protects us from potentially harmful environmental factors, such as infection-causing bacteria, the elements, and extremes in temperature. Our skin allows us to feel the sensations of pressure, pain, heat, and cold. It also can provide clues to internal disease. See Figure 1 of the appendix for a diagram of the skin.

SKIN AND HEALING

Skin cells constantly renew themselves in cell turnover cycles. Our epidermis, the outer layer of skin, is renewed approximately every month. The frequent growth of new skin cells and sloughing off of the old dead skin cells allows minor cuts and scrapes to heal as rapidly as they do. The state of one's overall health can significantly affect the ability of the skin to heal.

SKIN COLOR

There are all kinds of natural variations in human bodies. People differ in height and in the shape and size of their body parts. Another difference among humans is skin color, which can be varying hues of white, yellow, red, brown, and black. The color of each individual's skin ultimately depends upon his or her genetic makeup.

Skin color is determined by the pigment-producing cells in the epidermis called the melanocytes. Although skin color ranges from almost black to very pale, everyone has the same number of pigment-producing cells; it's the size and activity level of these cells that determine the color of a person's skin. Those with light skin have smaller, less active melanocytes compared to those with dark skin (with larger, more productive melanocytes). Melanocyte size is genetically determined, perhaps influenced through evolution of ancestral background, which may explain why people of African descent have darker skin. The

Teach your children to love and accept themselves.

melanocytes of people of African descent grew darker in order to protect against intense sun exposure, while the skin of Northern Europeans had less exposure to such intense sunlight.

The production of melanin is called melanogenesis, which determines a person's skin, hair, and eye color. How much or how little melanogenesis takes place is determined by the genes a child inherits from each birth parent and results in the diversity of human skin tones.

Skin color crosses perceived racial boundaries and social groups, so it is not possible (or sensitive to a person's culture or genetics) to attempt to define a person by his or her skin color. Judging someone by the color of his or her skin is a form of racism. A child with dark skin may be African American, African, Indian, Middle Eastern, Australian Aboriginal, Caribbean, Brazilian, or from any number of other geographical locations. Each individual, with his or her own unique skin color, is beautiful.

No skin color can be labeled "unattractive" or "bad". Historically, certain humans have judged or mistreated other humans, viewing them as inferior, based upon differences in religion, politics, ancestry, and social status, as well as skin color or other physical characteristics. Fortunately, modern concepts of tolerance and diversity are changing that. Whatever the color of your skin or your child's skin, every person can learn to appreciate and love his or her unique genetics and skin color. Teach your children to love and accept themselves, starting with their bodies, their physical selves, including their skin and hair.

Skin Types

THERE ARE TWO DIFFERENT WAYS to think about skin type. The first has to do with phototype, or the sensitivity of our skin to UV ray exposure. The Food and Drug Administration (FDA) and the American Academy of Dermatology (AAD) recognize six types of skin, based on photo or light sensitivity. [1,2]

The scale was invented to predict how patients would respond to light therapy for psoriasis and has since been used in many aspects of dermatology.

Table 1: Skin Types[3]

Type	Description of Skin Type and Examples	Does skin burn?	Ability to suntan
I	Very Light or Celtic	Often/Easily	Occasionally
II	Light	Usually/Easily	Sometimes
III	Darker European	Rarely	Usually
IV	Mediterranean, Olive, East Asian	Rarely	Often
V	Dark, Brown	Very rarely	May darken
VI	Very Dark	Extremely rarely	Naturally dark

Beyond differences in skin color (which may be a general indicator of UV exposure sensitivity) and skin phototype (which we can determine after sun exposure), we each have another variation in skin type. This has to do with whether our skin is dry, normal, oily, sensitive, or some combination of these. A baby's, child's, or teen's skin is always more sensitive than adult skin, as it is thinner and the sweat and sebaceous glands are less developed. Most children will display skin traits similar to their biological parents. You may not have information about your child's birth parents, so it is important for you to monitor your child's skin and skin care. No matter what color, phototype, or type of skin your

---

1 Fitzpatrick TB. The validity and practicality of sun-reactive skin types I through VI. Arch Dermatol. 1988.124:869-871.

2 Sunscreen drug products for over-the-counter human use (21CFR352). Food and Drug Administration. www.accessdata.fda.gov/scripts/cdrh/cfdocs/cfCFR/CFRSearch.cfm?CFRPart=352.

3 http://www.aad.org/media-resources/stats-and-facts/prevention-and-care/sunscreens

Our children learn to love themselves, including their physical appearance, when we teach them to do so.

child has, you should take care of and appreciate his or her skin and make sure they know that you appreciate it.

The purpose of this book is to help you learn to take good care of and maintain the health of your child's skin and hair. This nurturing is both physical and emotional. As part of this, avoid using or exposing your child to negative words and images regarding hair and skin. This may mean monitoring magazine and television media images and refusing to allow certain popular culture media to enter your home. Negative comments about your child's skin and hair will only upset your child and detract from his or her self-esteem. Our children learn to love themselves, including their physical appearance, when we teach them to do so. Show your children how special they are and how beautiful their skin is. Teach them that caring for their skin requires care, time, and effort and is important and worthwhile.

Set aside a time to "do skin care" with your child. Time spent caring for or teaching your child to care for his or her skin offers you an opportunity to talk with and nurture your child while you teach proper, loving self-care. Teaching your children to appreciate and love their skin is a way to teach them to appreciate and love themselves. Self-esteem is an important foundation for personal and professional success in life. Parental attitudes affect children's attitudes toward themselves and others.

Skin FAQs

CERTAIN QUESTIONS ABOUT SKIN CARE come up more frequently than any others. I have shared these commonly asked questions and their answers in this chapter. Adoptive parents often have a great many questions about their children's skin, especially when they do not have any birth family information or a medical history. Some frequently asked questions are:

1. *What kind of skin products (such as cleanser or moisturizer) should my child use?*

SKIN-CARE PRODUCTS

This depends on the condition of your child's skin (which can vary seasonally and geographically). Generally, skin-care products for infants and young children should be very emollient, moisturizing, and have little to no fragrance. Because the barrier function in young skin is not fully developed, products may assist in this function. Product choice will also vary seasonally. Choose cleansers that are gentle and creamy. In Chicago, we have very harsh winters and therefore need heavier, creamier products during those times. I always recommend moisturizers in a jar for winter. Often, you cannot put or keep enough moisture in the skin during this time of year. During the summer months, or in more humid environments, a lotion that is pumped or poured is a better choice. Generally the same cleanser and moisturizer can be used on the face and body for infants and young children. This should change once the hormones kick in and children become acne-prone, as heavier moisturizing products may worsen acne.

In lecturing to transcultural adoptive families, I often hear that their children's skin is very dry, yet they are hesitant to use heavier creams thought to be "too greasy." As a result, they don't use it on their child's skin and the problem continues. A heavy cream is exactly what this very dry skin needs. So, although it may be heavier than one which you would choose for yourself, remember, your child's skin is different than yours.

The purpose of using a moisturizer is to trap the moisture next to the skin and create a barrier/line of defense against outside environmental dangers, such as bacteria, yeast, etc. Applying these heavier creams is a wonderful opportunity to lovingly connect with your baby or your child by giving them a massage while applying the moisturizer.

It is important for your children not to be affected by your reaction to their need for certain skin-care products. Inexpert opinions (such as "This product is greasy") can give your child the wrong message. If a child sees you have a negative reaction to a product, they may believe you are having a negative reaction to them or their skin. Be careful to give your child positive, loving, and accepting messages about themselves.

2. How often should my child cleanse his or her skin?

CLEANSING

This depends on the age of the child and other conditions in the skin. Newborns and infants can be bathed daily or every two or three days if their skin is very sensitive. Starting in toddlerhood, bathing should become part of the nighttime getting-ready-for-bed routine. The nighttime routine is an opportunity to start teaching your child about proper skin care. Develop a skin-care regimen and a skin-care kit for your baby, child, or teen and use it (or teach them to use it). A child who is very active, plays outside a lot, or is involved in sports may need to bathe more frequently (whenever their skin gets dirty or sweaty) than a child who is less physically active. Teach your child to perform a skin-care routine, including bathing, moisturizing, and protecting the skin with sunscreen rather than just washing with hand soap.

3. Is dry skin a symptom of disease?

DRYNESS

Dry skin is common and not usually a symptom of disease, but it can be. Dry skin is often worse in the winter months in colder climates. First, eliminate anything that might be causing dry skin. Avoid long, hot baths with drying soap. Bubble baths are notorious for drying out the skin, although they are a favorite with toddlers. Bubble baths can be used as an occasional treat but should *not* be used on a regular basis. Look for bath products that contain some oil, such as Shea butter. Shorten the duration of the bath or shower if dry skin is an issue. Generally ten minutes is long enough to clean what needs to be cleaned. Moisturize, moisturize—if you are using moisturizer that pumps or pours, and the skin is still dry, change to a heavier jar moisturizer that you scoop to apply. The purpose of moisturizer is to trap moisture next to the skin; jar moisturizer will work better than other options. You may need to apply moisturizer as often as two or three times per day. Make sure that your home is well humidified.

If a child's dry skin doesn't respond to treatment, consult a dermatologist. Untreated dry skin can become itchy, inflamed, swollen, irritated, and red, and chronic scratching can cause small breaks in the skin, making the child more susceptible to infection.

4. Would a facial be good for my teenager?

FACIALS

I consider facials to be in the same category as massages. They are a treat for teens and adults, but not necessary if skin is properly cared for. A proper daily skin care regimen with appropriate products is more important than a periodic facial. Parents of tweens and teens ask this question hoping that a facial will prevent acne. Because many factors (hormonal, genetic, and habitual) contribute to acne, it is not preventable. Acne can be controlled; it cannot be prevented or cured. Facials can also be expensive. More important than teen facials is instruction in proper skin care, the use of appropriate products, and the use of acne medication if needed.

5. What do I do if my child has a rash?

RASHES

Rashes and other skin eruptions can have any number of causes. A rash could be caused by a chronic skin condition, such as eczema, and require medical management. Rashes may also be associated with fever, viral illness, medications, or other causes, so it is important to see a dermatologist for evaluation and treatment of a rash or other skin condition. A rash that is accompanied by a fever requires immediate medical care.

SUNSCREEN

6. *How old does my child need to be to use sunscreen?*

Ideally your infant will be at least six months old before you use sunscreen on him or her. Sensitive and delicate baby skin can be very damaged by sunburn, increasing the likelihood of skin cancer later in life. So if at all possible, avoid exposing a baby six months old or younger to the sun. If he or she must be in the sun, then I recommend an infant sunscreen product. A sunscreen with a minimum sun protection factor (SPF) of 30 is recommended and should be reapplied every two hours as these protective products break down in the sun. It is important to choose a product that says it is *broad spectrum* (with UVA and UVB coverage) and that contains one of the following compounds known to filter UV rays: zinc oxide, titanium dioxide, oxybenzone, ecamsule, or avobenzone. The use of sun protection should become habit. My kids know that before they go outside, they must put on their "suncream."

Clothing may also protect from the sun; there are several companies that make sun-protective clothing for adults and toddlers (you'll find their websites listed in the resource guide at the end of this book).

Make sure your stroller has a sunshade and your child is equipped with sunglasses and a hat, ideally a high-quality, protective sun hat made of sun-protective and UV-ray-blocking material. A sun hat and sun-protective clothing are especially important if your child is too young for sunscreen.

As mentioned earlier, even dark skin can burn. A family recently came to see me with questions about skin protection for their adopted daughter. The parents were Caucasian and understood why *they* needed sun protection yet mistakenly thought that their four-year-old from Guatemala did not need any sun protection because of her naturally dark skin. All skin can burn, and chronic sun damage will increase the risk of skin cancer regardless of skin color. Bob Marley died of a melanoma!

Getting Started—Basic Skin Care

HEALTHY SKIN STARTS WITH CLEAN SKIN, which should then be moisturized and protected. The skin products you use for your child or infant should be age- and skin-type-appropriate and gentle for the skin and body.

Cleanse your baby's face and body using a soft cloth and a gentle cleanser (see my list of suggested products at the back of this book). Baths should be no longer than five or ten minutes with tepid to warm water. Newborns cannot regulate their body temperature well, so it is not uncommon for newborn babies to shiver or for the skin to turn a bit blue when they have no clothes on. Keep this in mind when bathing or changing your infant. Minimize his or her exposure to cool air and keep the bathroom warmer than you normally would for yourself. If the skin does not return to its normal color, or if the child seems to constantly shiver, consult your child's pediatrician. Remove your baby from the water and bundle him or her up for warmth. In general, infants and toddlers need one more layer of clothing than adults do.

After cleansing the skin, liberally apply moisturizer to the entire body. Adult skin functions as a barrier between our internal organs and irritants of the outside world, but infant skin does not have this fully functioning barrier. Choose a moisturizer that protects the skin and seals in moisture. These are often a bit heavier in texture. One good one is Cetaphil Restoraderm. While applying moisturizer, take the time to give infants a full-body massage to help them to learn your loving touch. Newborn skin is often particularly dry and flaky. Full-body application of moisturizer with each diaper change can help significantly. Because newborns don't sweat very much, bathing every two to three days is sufficient.

Children under six months of age should have minimal or no sun exposure. Sun protection at this age means keeping your baby out of the sun and using broad-brimmed hats and a stroller shade. Sunscreen use generally begins at six months of age. Adjust your child's basic facial or body skin-care routine if he or she has a particular skin condition; read

The skin products you use for your child or infant should be age- and skin-type-appropriate.

about at-home treatments and when to seek medical treatment for a particular skin condition in the next section.

Taking care of one's skin is a learned behavior, and just like tooth brushing, should be incorporated into a daily hygiene routine and taught early. Teach your child to complete a daily facial skin care regimen to cleanse, moisturize, and protect, each morning and night. Make them aware that they will need to wash again after play, athletics, or exercise, when they can get sweaty and dirty. Until your child reaches adolescence, the same products can be used on the face and body. Once the hormones kick in and skin becomes more acne-prone, he or she will need different products for the face and for the body. Be certain to explain the difference between cleansing the body and the facial skin to your child. We know that increased sun exposure and frequent sunburns as a child significantly increases the lifetime risk of skin cancer, regardless of skin color, so teaching your child proper sun protection habits at a young age is crucial to a lifetime of good skin health.

Make sure you practice what you preach since children are wonderful imitators of behavior. Application of broad-spectrum sunscreen with minimum SPF 15 should be part of the daily routine for everyone in your household and, because we know that UV rays are carcinogens, by all means teach them that sunbathing and tanning is dangerous to their health, regardless of skin color.

It is said that repetition is the mother of learning. As your child's first guide to life, you may need to explain facial and body skin care to them on more than one occasion (depending upon his or her age and level of comprehension). Below is a step-by-step guide to caring for your child's facial skin.

Caring for Your Child's Facial Skin

Grab your child's skin-care kit and get out your child's facial products. Put all three products (cleanser, moisturizer, and sunscreen) where they will be handy. Get a soft washcloth and a hand towel. Depending upon the age of your child, you will either perform the facial skin care routine or supervise it. Make the routine fun so your kids will enjoy it.

Teach your child to complete a daily facial skin care regimen to cleanse, moisturize, and protect, each morning and night.

STEP 1

Step 1—Cleansing your child's skin

With warm/tepid water on a damp washcloth, apply a small amount of mild cleanser and gently wash your child's face. You can use a clean, damp cotton ball or the corner of a clean, damp washcloth, with no cleanser, to carefully wipe each eyelid. Avoid scrubbing. Carefully wash the neck or other creases where drool and food may collect. Pat the skin dry with a towel. There is no need to wipe the skin completely dry, as a bit of water on the surface will be trapped by the skin cream, creating more hydration for the skin.

STEP 2

Step 2—Moisturizing your child's skin

After your child's skin is clean but still a little bit moist, liberally apply (or have your child apply) a moisturizer. Remember to choose a product in a jar for winter and pump or pour for summer. These specifically chosen moisturizers will seal in the skin's natural moisture.

STEP 3

Step 3—Protecting your child's skin

The amount of sun protection needed depends on how much of the body needs to be covered. Adults generally need a full ounce of sun protection (about the amount to fill a shot glass) for a full-body application. Toddlers should use about half of this amount. When in doubt, apply more. Cover the areas of your child's skin that will be exposed to the sun's rays. (If your child is younger than six months, don't use sunscreen and keep him or her out the sun if at all possible.)

In order for the sun-protective ingredients to become active, they should be applied twenty minutes before outdoor activities. Remember to reapply after two hours and after water activities or heavy sweating. Finding a product with the proper ingredients as well as the proper texture may require some experimentation. Remember, some physical blockers (for example, titanium dioxide and zinc oxide) are rather pasty and may not rub in well on dark skin tones. This is not a reason to skip sunscreen. Choose one that rubs in nicely and does not leave an obvious white or chalky film. You may need to try several in order to find one that will nearly disappear. As long as the product contains SPF 30 or greater, has broad spectrum UVA/UVB protection, and is reapplied every two hours, the choice of product is up to you!

Quick Tips for Caring for your Child's Skin

- Establish a facial and body skin-care routine for your child or teen.

- Make your child's self-care routines enjoyable to create lifetime habits.

- Avoid using skin-care products with harsh or irritating ingredients.

- Monitor your child's skin, paying special attention to moles and warts.

- Monitor and protect your child's sensitive skin from the sun, heat, and cold.

- Keep well-baby and well-child appointments. Many skin conditions can be treated and resolved, especially if they are discovered early.

In general, you can protect and maintain the beauty and health of your child's or teen's skin with the simple routines described in this section. However, some children have special skin-care needs. If your youngster has a particular skin issue, condition, or disease, it is likely to affect his or her daily skin-care routine, and you should adjust the routine accordingly. Certain skin issues and conditions may require special, perhaps even medicated, face or body products. The following sections of this book describe specific skin-care conditions, as well as their symptoms, causes, and recommended treatments.

SPECIAL NOTE

Special note on facial cleansing and acne:

Some parents come to my office seeking treatment for their tween's or teen's acne. Very commonly, the parent insists the child has acne because he or she is not washing his or her face frequently enough. There are many factors that contribute to acne (see the acne section for more detailed and specific information), and while washing one's face is important, it is not a cure for acne. For adolescents and preteens, acne is primarily hormonal. Although it is not avoidable, acne is treatable. So try not to blame your child for things that are out of his or her control. The teen years are challenging enough without additional emotional pressure and negative experiences. I have seen too many teen patients embarrassed and ashamed when their parents wrongly insist that the teen's acne is his or her own fault.

Skin-Care Kit

MAKE A SKIN-CARE KIT to make your child's daily facial skin-care regimen easier. Be sure to explain the purpose and use of the skin-care kit and everything inside it (if your child can understand). Taking the time to focus on and enjoy this creative self-care activity with your child or teen will make it a pleasant bonding experience. Let your child make some of his or her own choices, when appropriate, to help you create the kit.

Stay free of irritating chemicals/ingredients such as parabens, sulfates, synthetic fragrances, artificial colors, petrochemicals, and phthalates.

Include facial skin care products in your child's kit that are age- and skin-type-specific, as natural as possible, and free of any potentially irritating chemicals or other ingredients (such as parabens, sulfates, synthetic fragrances, artificial colors, petrochemicals, and phthalates). A washcloth is a gentle way to cleanse, massage, and assist the natural exfoliation process (in which skin cells on the surface shed every couple of weeks). Pick up washcloths in colors that your child likes; you can keep one in the kit and keep the others with your linens.

Get a medium-sized box, preferably waterproof with a handle, to organize and carry the skin care kit. Let your child decorate or choose the box himself to give him a sense of ownership and increase the likelihood that he will use and enjoy it. Include the following items in your child's kit:

- Cleanser
- Moisturizer
- Sunscreen
- SPF lip balm
- Soft washcloth
- Cotton balls (or pads)

After pulling together these items, sit down with your child to walk through his or her regimen. Make this time a loving experience. While you wash, moisturize, and protect your child's skin, be sure to tell him or her how beautiful he or she is. Talk about how much you enjoy taking care of him or her.

Skin Issues from A to Z

While many skin conditions may be chronic, they are generally treatable and controllable.

IT IS ESSENTIAL TO MONITOR YOUR CHILD'S SKIN. Perhaps you have access to the medical history of his or her biological family and are aware of familial skin issues to watch out for, but you may not. Your child may have hereditary issues or sensitivities of which you are unaware or with which you are unfamiliar. Careful observation of your child's skin may alert you to a condition, serious or not, that requires treatment.

Skin issues are not uncommon in infants, young children, and teens, and while many of these conditions may be chronic, they are generally treatable and controllable. For example, we cannot cure eczema, but we do know what may make it worse, which treatments will alleviate the symptoms, and what skin-care regimen will keep skin healthy. Because the skin is the largest organ and visible to the outside world, skin conditions may affect your growing child's self-esteem. Some skin conditions can be more serious or take longer to resolve, and a rare few, such as pediatric skin cancer, are quite serious. Use the index of this book if you suspect your child has a skin condition and consult your dermatologist if you have concerns.

Dry Skin (Xerosis Cutis)

DRY SKIN IS QUITE COMMON. The sebaceous glands in our skin normally produce adequate amounts of oil or lipids to lubricate the skin, but any number of factors can lead to abnormally dry skin or xerosis cutis. Darker skin may look "ashy" when it is very dry.

Dry Skin Symptoms

SYMPTOMS

- Itching
- Redness
- Dullness
- Flakiness
- Roughness
- Fissures/Cracks (may be deep/bleed)

Dry Skin Causes

CAUSES

Skin gets dry when natural oils, or lipids, and water is lacking. Environmental exposure is the primary offender and source of dry skin conditions. Our skin tends to be driest when humidity levels are low. Air conditioners, room heaters, furnaces, and stoves all affect humidity levels and can cause dry skin. Also, frequent bathing with hot or very warm water and the use of certain soaps and skin cleansers can affect the skin's lipid barriers and strip the skin of its natural moisture, as can frequent swimming (especially in chlorine-treated water).

Dry Skin Treatment

TREATMENT

In most cases, a doctor's visit is not required to successfully take care of dry skin. Dry skin responds well to over-the-counter remedies and lifestyle changes. Recommended treatment for dry skin includes:

- Shorten baths or showers to ten minutes or less.
- Turn down the water temperature. The bath or shower

should be warm, not hot. A good rule of thumb is that if steam appears on the mirror, it's too hot!

- Use gentle, non-fragranced cleansers (no deodorant soaps or bubble baths).

- Heavy-up the moisturizer. Switch to a jar (scoop) moisturizer in the winter. Heavier moisturizers trap moisture next to the skin.

- Moisturize more than once a day, such as in the morning and at night. Infants may need heavier moisturizer with each diaper change. Send school-aged children to school with a moisturizer to apply during the day if they get itchy.

- Adjust the humidity in the home or consider a humidifier in the bedroom.

- Make sure the child takes a bath or shower soon after swimming to remove the chlorine, then liberally apply a heavier moisturizer.

- Use gentle fabrics next to skin—the first layer should preferably be cotton.

WHEN TO SEE A DERMATOLOGIST

Dry skin is itchy and may crack. Constant scratching can create micro tears that disrupt the protective barrier function of the skin. Once this is compromised, the risk of infection increases. Most dry skin is seasonal and controllable. If dry skin doesn't improve with at-home treatment, see a dermatologist. Dry skin can be a symptom of other medical conditions such as eczema, diabetes, and thyroid problems, which require individualized medical evaluation and treatment.

Atopic Dermatitis (Eczema)

ATOPIC DERMATITIS OR ECZEMA IS A VERY COMMON skin condition. It is often genetically determined and is seen more commonly in families who also have the following conditions: hay fever, sinus problems, asthma, and seasonal allergies. If anyone in the genetic family has any of these conditions then everyone is prone to developing any of these conditions. This is very important to understand and underscores why extended birth family history is helpful.

Eczema is characterized by irritation and inflammation affecting the epidermis, or outermost skin layer. It causes a rash that is often itchy. When the skin is scratched, a crust or scabs may form in the area. Once your child's skin barrier is broken, the chance of a skin infection increases. It's not uncommon for children with eczema to have localized skin infections as well as eczema. The condition can cause post inflammatory hyperpigmentation (darkening of the skin), especially in children with darker skin tones. This can take months or years to fade away, or it may be permanent.

Eczema Skin Symptoms

SYMPTOMS

- Dry skin patches, often on the face, scalp, hands, feet, elbows, backs of the knees and/or on the wrists, neck, chest, and ankles

- Itching (mild to severe)

- Open areas that may weep/ooze and then crust over

- Skin may thicken in areas of constant scratching

- Scratching exacerbates the rash (this is often referred to as "the itch-scratch cycle": the more you itch the more you scratch)

Causes of Eczema

Although the exact cause of eczema is still unknown, contributing factors may include immune system dysfunction and genetic predisposition. While eczema is not caused by stress, stress can certainly exacerbate the condition. These stressors can be both emotional and physical. It is not uncommon for eczema to flare when a child experiences a stressor such as a cold, an ear infection, a new sibling, a new school or any other situation that may be stressful. Stress, whether it is physical or emotional, puts a strain on the immune system and makes us less able to handle certain conditions. Think about the times you have gotten the flu or a cold (both viruses that take advantage of lowered immune status). These times likely coincided with your feeling overworked, run-down, and tired, all signs of a taxed immune system.

Eczema Treatment

People with eczema have itching that can at times be unrelenting and severe. Telling your child to stop scratching is unlikely to do the trick. Chronic scratching can lead to thickening of the skin, which is called lichenification. Successful treatment of eczema often involves interrupting the "itch-scratch" cycle with intermittent use of prescription-strength medication.

Relationship Between Skin, Immune Function, and Stress

Skin health, stress, and immune function are related. People who've been under greater-than-average physical or emotional stress, including neglect, abuse, chronic illness, or alcohol or drug withdrawal, may have compromised immune systems and resultant exacerbation of existing skin conditions such as eczema.

TREATMENT

Recommended Eczema Treatment

- Treat exacerbating causes (ear infections, asthma flare-ups, etc.).

- Consider seeing an allergist for prick testing to determine if environmental or food allergies are present.

- Address emotional stresses or concerns your child may be experiencing. (Children may not be able to easily communicate their emotional stressors. Talk to your child about likely problems—academic, emotional, or otherwise.)

- Keep showers/baths short (no longer than ten minutes) and warm (not hot). You can use a bathroom egg timer with older children to keep their showers within recommended limits.

- Use gentle, non-irritating, non-deodorant soaps.

- Use heavier emollients (jar), more than once a day, as a barrier protectant or for their skin repair properties (Cera Ve, Aveeno Eczema Therapy Moisturizing Cream, and Cetaphil Restoraderm Skin Restoring Moisturizer).

- Avoid dryer sheets, which deposit an irritating film of fragrance in the clothing.

- Use fragrance-, dye- and additive-free laundry detergent (such as Dreft, Cheer Free and Gentle, or All Free Clear).

- Increase humidity in the home (a humidifier in your child's room at night is recommended).

- Take note of any foods that make the eczema worse and have your child avoid them (citrus and dairy may be offenders).

- Have your child rinse off and moisturize well after being in a pool or the ocean; salt and chlorine can be very drying to the skin.

WHEN TO SEE A DERMATOLOGIST

Consult an expert if there is a known genetic family history of eczema or if your child has rashes that don't improve with the suggestions above. Eczema is a chronic condition that can persist through adulthood. For young children and infants, the itching is too difficult to bear without some kind of treatment. Itching can become so severe that it interferes with the ability to sleep or distracts a child from normal activities (including school). Scratching can worsen the condition; children may scratch until the skin bleeds, which can cause infection. It is essential to treat this condition.

A dermatologist can further advise you about what to do and what to avoid as well as prescribe medications (steroids, immune modulator creams, or antihistamines) that can alleviate symptoms and improve or control the condition. Antibiotics may be necessary for related skin infections.

Keratosis Pilaris

KERATOSIS PILARIS, ALSO KNOWN AS KP, is sometimes called "chicken skin." Common in children and young adults, this condition occurs when keratin, a protein in the skin, forms a hard plug in the hair follicles of dead skin cells.

Keratosis pilaris generally forms on the outer areas of the upper arms (triceps) as well as on the thighs, upper back, and cheeks. KP is often associated with children who have a personal or genetic atopic history. KP on the cheeks is generally outgrown whereas KP on the arms, thighs, and upper back tends to persist. KP also tends to improve with humidity in the summer and worsen in cold winter environments.

Keratosis Pilaris Symptoms

- Red bumps/rough skin texture on the cheek, upper outer arm, thigh, and upper back. Skin may feel like sandpaper.

- Itching (especially in winter or in low-humidity climates).

- Coiled or ingrown hairs trapped in hair follicles.

Keratosis Pilaris Causes

Keratosis pilaris is an inherited condition which is thought to occur in as much as 40 percent or more of the world's population. It is often seen in patients who have a personal or genetic family atopic history (hay fever, eczema, sinus problems, asthma).

Keratosis Pilaris Treatment

In most cases, KP is treated for its appearance or for extreme itching or other symptoms. Keratosis pilaris can't be cured but instead the symptoms are treated and the condition may improve. KP treatments often include:

- Use of moisturizers or emollients to decrease dryness/redness.

- Use of a mild exfoliant product with urea or lactic acid to soften hard, crusty skin. (I recommend avoiding use of this product with infants and young children due to the irritation of the exfoliant.)

- Use of topical retinoids to minimize the appearance of red bumps, although topical retinoids may be too irritating for already sensitive skin.

WHEN TO SEE A DERMATOLOGIST

See a dermatologist to get a proper diagnosis if you suspect your infant, child, or teen has KP. Treatment for KP is not necessary, since the condition is harmless. Symptom management could be important for cosmetic reasons or to help your child deal with very itchy bumps. Certain treatments may not be recommended for infants or young children. Do not attempt to treat your infant or child without consulting an expert for diagnosis and treatment guidance, as many over-the-counter or at-home remedies can exacerbate this condition. KP treatment is generally ongoing, as beneficial results are usually temporary. Some patients, naturally, respond better to KP treatment than others do.

Intertrigo/Diaper Rash

INTERTRIGO IS AN INFLAMMATORY REACTION between folds of the skin in areas that rub against each other and are moist. Intertrigo is often commonly seen in babies under the chin, in the creases of the arms and knees, and in the diaper area. All children can get this rash; however, because it is often seen in areas where there is skin on skin contact as well as moisture and heat, it is more often seen in children (and adults) with a few rolls of fat. It will also get worse when babies start to teethe because of the constant drool. Once the child starts to walk, which should decrease the skin rolls, and there is less drool, much of this will resolve. Frequent rubbing of the skin can lead to skin breakdown, which will then increase the risk of localized bacterial infection.

Intertrigo Symptoms

SYMPTOMS

- Reddened, moist, and shiny skin
- Scaly or chafed skin
- Blistering or broken skin
- Oozing
- Itching/sore skin

Intertrigo Causes

CAUSES

Intertrigo—diaper rash—is caused by skin breakdown in very moist skin areas.

Intertrigo Treatment

TREATMENT

Intertrigo is treated by eliminating the circumstances which are creating the condition and related symptoms. In most cases, intertrigo symptoms improve when you:

- Keep the skin area clean and dry. If possible, take the diapers off just after a diaper change and let the area air out. Make sure to clean area under the chin and diaper area well after each feeding or diaper change with a damp cloth.

- You may want to discontinue baby wipes during treatment and use a soft washcloth with mild soap.

- Use an over-the-counter barrier cream, such as a zinc cream product, and apply to the folds of the skin and under the chin, wherever symptomatic, several times daily.

Treatment of Intertrigo-Related Viral, Bacterial, or Fungal Infections

Once you've eliminated or minimized, as much as possible, the moisture and friction creating the skin inflammation, or intertrigo, it is essential to treat any related viral-, bacterial-, or fungus-related issues. Moist, damaged skin is extremely susceptible to secondary infection due to the growth of microorganisms which should be treated with specific, often prescription, medication.

WHEN TO SEE A DERMATOLOGIST

Have a dermatologist evaluate intertrigo/diaper rash and recommend treatment, especially if it does not resolve with the above suggestions. Your dermatologist can diagnose and treat any associated secondary infections with appropriate prescription medications.

Acne: Neonatal and Infant

NEONATAL OR NEWBORN BABY ACNE is fairly common, particularly among infant boys. Like adolescent and other types of acne, it is an inflammatory skin reaction brought on by hormones (which are, in the case of newborn acne, passed from mother to baby before birth). Neonatal acne often shows up in baby's first few weeks of life and usually clears up, without scarring, in a few months. Newborn acne, in rare cases, may be severe and persist for months. It is often more severe in infant boys.

Neonatal (Newborn) Acne Symptoms

SYMPTOMS

- Appears in first few days, sometimes months, of baby's life.

- Plugged pores or pustules on cheeks or chin, eyelids, upper chest, or neck skin of a newborn baby.

- Usually improves and clears up within weeks or a few months without treatment.

Neonatal Acne Causes

CAUSES

Neonatal acne is caused when testosterone increases, in male and female infants, because hormones are passed to a baby from the mother before birth. The hormones stimulate sebaceous gland production, and they enlarge and produce oil and may then plug the pores of your newborn baby's skin.

Neonatal Acne Treatment

Often newborn acne resolves within a few days or months without treatment. In most cases, newborn acne symptoms improve when you:

- Gently cleanse your baby's skin (removing all food products).

- Minimize use of heavy emollient products on the face.

- Avoid use of over-the-counter acne medications, as they are too irritating for delicate baby skin.

WHEN TO SEE A DERMATOLOGIST

A dermatologist can treat your new baby's severe acne and provide ongoing care, including prescription of mild topical creams. If your baby has an olive or darker skin tone, he or she is at greater risk for post-inflammatory hyperpigmentation (dark spots where acne lesions were). Consult your dermatologist about treatment to ensure the health of your new baby's skin.

Infantile Acne

INFANTILE ACNE IS A MORE SERIOUS TYPE OF BABY ACNE. Infantile acne may linger for months or years. Like other types of acne, it is an inflammatory skin reaction brought on by hormones (as with neonatal acne, the hormones were passed from mother to child before birth). Infantile acne often shows up when your baby is about three months old. It generally clears up, without scarring, in the first year of life but sometimes persists and is severe.

Infantile Acne Symptoms

SYMPTOMS

- Appears when baby is three to six months old
- More common in boys than in girls
- Plugged pores (whiteheads/blackheads) on face, upper chest, or neck skin
- Inflamed pimples/pustules or yellow papules
- May be severe and last for several years

PATIENT STORY

I often see my infantile acne patients when they are the first child in the family and either 1) family photos are coming up, or 2) the grandmothers are coming to town.

Infantile Acne Causes

CAUSES

The cause of infantile acne is unknown but is not thought to be hormonal. Children who have severe infantile acne may have acne in puberty.

Infantile Acne Treatment

Often infantile acne resolves within a few months though it can take years. In most cases, infantile acne symptoms improve when you:

- Gently cleanse your child's skin (keeping it clear of food debris).

- Use only water or the mildest of pediatric cleansers to clean the skin.

- Avoid picking at the whiteheads or blackheads on your child's skin.

- Use dermatologist-prescribed topical acne products in severe cases.

WHEN TO SEE A DERMATOLOGIST

A dermatologist can treat your child's infantile acne and provide ongoing care (including prescription of mild topical creams). As with newborn acne, avoid use of over-the-counter acne products designed for teens. If your child or toddler has or develops other signs of puberty, he or she should be tested for medical conditions which have abnormally high levels of puberty hormones as a symptom. Consult your dermatologist to ensure the continued health and beauty of your young child's skin. Adolescent acne, a different condition from either infant or neonatal acne, is discussed in the next section of this book.

Acne

ACNE IS A COMMON INFLAMMATORY SKIN REACTION with plugged pores and inflamed pustules, which affects teens at the onset of adolescence and may persist through adulthood. It is the most common skin condition in the US and generally affects the face, back, and chest. Untreated acne may permanently scar your teenager's face and self-esteem. It is very important to treat your teenage or tween child's acne.

Acne Symptoms

Symptoms

- Plugged pores (whiteheads/blackheads)
- Pus-filled lumps or cysts
- Pimples/pustules
- Deeper lumps (nodules)

Acne Causes

Causes

Acne is caused when hormones increase during puberty and sebaceous gland production is stimulated. Sebaceous glands enlarge and increase oil production, which may then plug the pores of your child's skin and cause breakouts.

Acne Treatment

Treatment

Contrary to myth, adolescent acne is not the result of your child's failure to clean his or her skin or the result of a poor diet. Certain foods may aggravate acne—your child should avoid eating those foods if you observe worsening of acne. Acne often flares during periods of stress; such stressful periods may include exam time, before the menstrual cycle, or emotional times in your teenager or tween's life. Teen years are often difficult enough as children try to "find themselves." This period may be made more difficult with any unresolved adoption issues, such as knowledge of birth parent identity.

A dermatologist can treat both acne and acne scars (with microdermabrasion, laser, or chemical peels). Patients with darker skin tones are at greater risk for post-inflammatory hyperpigmentation (dark spots from acne lesions). Dark spots often take longer to treat; it is essential to get acne under control to minimize scarring and discoloration risk. In most cases, acne symptoms improve when you have your child:

- Use a gentle cleanser each night (removing all facial products).

- Use appropriate acne medications, either over-the-counter or, when these do not improve the condition, prescription products.

- Use noncomedogenic and nonacnegenic facial products.

- Avoid using heavy products on the face (body lotion and creams) at puberty.

- Be sure to clean skin soon after gym class, sports, and workouts.

WHEN TO SEE A DERMATOLOGIST

A dermatologist can treat teenage acne and prescribe hormonal, topical, or oral antibiotic treatments as well as acne surgery, microdermabrasion, laser, chemical peels, injections of corticosteroids for large nodules, or even photodynamic therapy. Teens with acne may be noncompliant or want instant results. A dermatologist can treat and guide your teen by teaching proper skin care and managing expectations.

Seborrheic Dermatitis
(Dandruff/Cradle Cap)

SEBORRHEIC DERMATITIS IS A COMMON CONDITION affecting people of all ethnic backgrounds. It affects hair-bearing areas of the body, most commonly the scalp, but may also affect the ears, eyebrows, and sides of the nose. On a baby's scalp, seborrheic dermatitis is called cradle cap. The form seen in teens and adults is dandruff (*read about this in part two of this book*).

Seborrheic Dermatitis Symptoms

SYMPTOMS

- Reddened (inflamed) hair-bearing skin
- Scaly patches of scalp skin (which may be crusty)
- Dandruff (yellow or white flakes)
- Itching (or sore) skin

Seborrheic Dermatitis Causes

CAUSES

The cause of seborrheic dermatitis appears to include sebaceous gland (skin oil) overproduction and an overgrowth of the yeast *Mallassezia furfur*. Stress, a weakened immune system, genetic predisposition, and hormonal fluctuations can all exacerbate the condition. The condition may be lifelong. There may also be seasonal fluctuation with the condition worsening in the winter months.

Seborrheic Dermatitis Treatment

TREATMENT

In most cases, seborrheic dermatitis improves with prescription antifungal creams and shampoos. Severe cases may benefit from the use of mild- to moderate-strength topical steroid creams or ointments for a short period of time. Long-term use of topical steroids can thin the skin and lighten dark skin, so use of steroid products should be supervised by a dermatologist.

PATIENT STORY: OVER-WASHING

I recently saw a family in the office who brought their nine-year-old adopted daughter in for dandruff/seborrheic dermatitis. The parents are Caucasian and their daughter is African American. They had seen another dermatologist several months prior who had given them a prescription dandruff shampoo and advised her to wash her hair every day. The parents followed these instructions for several weeks and noticed their daughter's scalp becoming increasingly dry. While the child did have seborrheic dermatitis, she was now over-washing her hair, which caused excessive dryness. I suggested she wash her hair every 7-10 days with the prescription medicated shampoo, but follow it with a second shampoo more specific for her tightly coiled hair. This would add more moisture followed by a detangling leave-in conditioner and her regular gentle styling.

The family returned several weeks later with the seborrheic dermatitis under control and the child's hair in much better condition. Generally, the curlier the hair, the less frequently you need to wash it. Very straight hair (Caucasian, Asian) should be washed every 1-3 days; wavy hair (Hispanic, bi-racial hair) every 3-5 days; and tightly coiled/curly hair every 7-10 days.

WHEN TO SEE A DERMATOLOGIST

Have a dermatologist evaluate your child's seborrheic dermatitis and prescribe treatment. Keep in mind this is a chronic condition that may fluctuate seasonally and with stress. Your dermatologist should recommend ways to manage this persistent issue. Topical medications come in a variety of textures (solutions, creams, and ointments), selected based on the area where it will be applied. Antifungal shampoos are often suggested. However, all medicated shampoos can be drying, especially to curly hair. Care must be taken not to over-wash curly hair to avoid breakage. (See the next section for further hair-care information.)

Skin Infection

It is important to protect skin, because although our skin is generally self-healing, any break or opening in the skin may get infected.

SKIN INFECTIONS ARE NOT UNCOMMON, especially in children who may accidentally scrape or cut the surface of their skin while playing or scratching, if they have a condition such as eczema that causes them to scratch frequently. It is important to protect skin, because although our skin is generally self-healing, any break or opening (including blisters that burst) in the skin may get infected. Very dry skin may even crack and put the skin at risk for infection. Different types of bacteria and fungus, as well as viruses, can infect human skin. Common skin infections include folliculitis, impetigo, cellulitis, and staph. Some skin infections are caused by waterborne bacteria. Symptoms of a skin infection include irritation, rashes, bumps, or blisters. Some skin is more sensitive than others and more susceptible to infection.

Prevent or reduce the likelihood of skin infections by encouraging your child to protect his or her skin. If your child has a cut, abrasion, or other wound, teach them to clean the area, apply an over-the-counter product to prevent infection, and cover the area with a Band-Aid or bandage. Make sure there are no exposed tags or seams in your child's clothing to cause irritation; pay particular attention to shoe fit so they do not rub and cause friction blisters. Some types of skin infection can be quite aggressive and hard to treat. It is easiest to prevent most skin infections rather than get them and then treat them. Any skin infection that does not improve with simple wound care or is accompanied by fever, swelling, or spreading should receive immediate medical attention.

Moles

MOLES ARE *MELANOCYTIC NEVI. Congenital nevi* are moles that are present at birth and have an increased risk of becoming atypical or cancerous during one's lifetime. Skin cancer can and does occur in children regardless of skin color. First-degree relatives of patients with melanoma have an increased risk of developing melanoma in their lifetime. Knowing birth parent medical history can be very important; however, it is not always available. It is not uncommon to develop moles from infancy until the early twenties; however, moles should be observed for any changes in color, size, or behavior. Exposure to sunlight can cause moles to darken, which is why it is imperative sun protection begin early and be consistent regardless of skin color or ethnic background.

Mole Symptoms

SYMPTOMS

- Brown or black (but can be blue, pinkish, or even yellow)
- Round, flat, oval, or raised
- Generally small and regular in shape
- Hair sometimes grows from a mole
- Generally benign (changes in a mole may indicate melanoma)

Mole Causes

CAUSES

Moles are a made up of nevus cells and a pigment cell malformation. They are genetically determined. Generally, moles don't require treatment unless they are suspicious, atypical, or have changed.

Mole Treatment

Moles require removal only if they are suspicious, atypical, or have changed. Removal of moles by laser surgery is controversial since lasers cause tissue destruction and leave nothing for pathologic diagnosis. Moles that require treatment should be biopsied, followed by complete surgical removal if indicated.

Mole Observation:

A—Asymmetry: if you cut the lesion in half, both sides should equal each other, if not, they are asymmetrical.

B—Borders: irregular borders.

C—Color: more than one color.

D—Diameter bigger than the eraser of a pencil: approximately 6mm.

E—Evolving/changing moles or NEW moles.

Keep in mind that these are guidelines for evaluating a mole. Any of the above changes in a mole should be brought to your dermatologist's attention.

Warts

WARTS ARE HIGHLY CONTAGIOUS and common noncancerous skin growths caused by human papilloma virus (HPV). Warts which can occur in any area of the body are usually not painful except for plantar warts on the bottom (or plantar) of the foot. Warts are generally passed from body-to-body contact. Your child might contract warts from a caregiver who touches them who has warts on their hands. If you or other caregivers have hand warts, please let your pediatrician know, as a child with warts in the genital area may raise the suspicion of sexual abuse.

Wart Symptoms

SYMPTOMS

- Flesh-colored bumps which often have a crusty surface.
- Round, flat, oval, or raised (and often rough to the touch).
- Generally do not hurt (except for plantar warts on the foot soles).

Wart Causes

CAUSES

Warts are caused by a form of the human papilloma virus (HPV).

Wart Treatment

TREATMENT

Treatment of warts is recommended, since they are highly contagious. Children who pick at their warts can spread them to other areas of their body, to their siblings, their playmates, and/or to their parents. Treatments which your dermatologist may provide include an at-home salicylic acid gel/solution (over-the-counter) treatment. Do not use on infants or young children without consulting a physician first, as these can be too irritating to delicate young skin.   In-office dermatologic treatments include:

- Cryotherapy—or freezing (may be painful)
- Electrosurgery—or burning (may be painful)

- Canthardin—causes wart to blister, destroying it; can be removed

- Peeling—various topical treatments applied daily

- Laser—can be used to treat/destroy certain warts

- Immunotherapy—using the body's immune system

- Topical prescription medication

Because warts are viral, once the virus has entered the system the child will always have the propensity to develop warts throughout his or her lifetime. Warts may develop in times of stress, when the immune system functioning is lowered.

WHEN TO SEE A DERMATOLOGIST

A dermatologist can identify whether a growth on your infant or child is actually a wart. Additionally, warts may require a combined treatment approach; warts may not respond to a single treatment and can sometimes be difficult to get rid of. Evaluation and treatment by a dermatologist is recommended.

Molluscum Contagiosum

MOLLUSCUM CONTAGIOSUM (MOLLUSCA) IS A VIRAL SKIN INFECTION. Like warts, they are caused by a virus and are contagious. Considered benign, they often appear in arm or groin folds, on the chest, stomach, and buttocks, in clusters, or on the face and eyelids.

Molluscum Contagiosum Symptoms

SYMPTOMS

- Flesh-colored, firm pink, or pearly (dome-shaped) nodules/growths
- May redden and become inflamed or raised
- Can appear shiny with a center indentation/white core

PATIENT STORY

I once had a family with four children who had molluscum contagiosum. It took over a year to clear the family of molluscum as the children repeatedly spread the lesions through play and bath-time, continually reinfecting each other.

Molluscum Contagiosum Causes

CAUSES

Molluscum contagiosum are caused by a poxvirus and a person may catch them from clothing or a swimsuit, or body-to-body contact with another person. Children with other skin conditions such as eczema are more prone to developing them.

Molluscum Contagiosum Treatment

Molluscum contagiosum will eventually resolve untreated, but since they are highly contagious, treatment is recommended. Treatments which your dermatologist may provide (some of which may be painful) include an at-home topical retinoid (available by prescription) or an antiviral application.

In-office dermatologic treatments:

- Cryotherapy—freezing with liquid nitrogen
- Electrocautery—electric needle cauterization
- Cantheradin—application of a topical blistering solution

Keep in mind that any destructive method of treating molluscum contagiosum may also destroy pigment producing melanocytes in brown skin which may leave lighter or darker spots in the treatment area.

WHEN TO SEE A DERMATOLOGIST

A dermatologist can treat or recommend at-home treatment and should be consulted if you think your child has mollusca.

Birthmarks

BIRTHMARKS ARE COMMON IN BABIES. Some babies are born with birthmarks; others develop them in the first few weeks of life. Newborn birthmarks are categorized as pigmented, vascular, or resulting from abnormal development. Birthmarks may be concerning for new parents. I recommend that you consult with a dermatologist after your child is born, or if you've recently adopted, as soon as you learn that your child has a birthmark. Congenital *melanocytic nevi* are moles that are present at birth. Some birthmarks aren't easy to identify. Certain birthmarks have malignant potential. All birthmarks, like any skin condition, should be monitored.

Types of Birthmarks

Pigmented Types
Mole (Congenital melanocytic nevus)

- Café au lait spot

- Mongolian spot (dermal melanocytosis)

Vascular Types

- Macular stain or stork bite (*Nevus flammeus nuchae*)

- Strawberry mark (hemangioma)

- Port-wine stain (*Nevus flammeus*)

Vascular Birthmark

A macular stain is the most common vascular birthmark. If they are located on the forehead, eyelids, upper lip, or nose, macular stains may be called "angel's kisses." If the marks are on the back of the neck, where the stork of myth might have carried the child by the back of the neck in its beak when the baby was delivered to the parents, they may be called "stork bites." Angel's kisses often fade over time; stork bites may remain for up to 25 percent of children.

Hermangioma

A hemangioma is a vascular birthmark that results when extra blood vessels group together into a dense configuration. Sometimes called a "strawberry mark," this usually starts out as a reddish or reddish-pink discoloration of the skin, most often on a child's scalp, face, or neck. Common in girls and premature babies, the mark can appear at birth but generally isn't observed until the first few weeks after a baby is born. A child can have more than one mark; the odds of multiple discolorations increase if the child was part of a multiple birth.

A hemangioma can sometimes become sore or ulcerated, which could be painful or susceptible to infection. If that happens, it is important to take your child to the dermatologist and have the area treated. Hemangiomas in functional areas of the body, such as the genitals or rectum, or near the ear, nose, or mouth, should be watched closely and treated if growth of the hemangioma may compromise function of these important areas. A hemangioma should not generally bleed unless it has been traumatized or injured.

Other vascular types of birthmark include stork bite and port-wine stain. A port-wine stain (*Nevus flammeus*) is permanent and will not fade on its own. However, it can be treated. Port-wine stains are often associated with more serious medical conditions, such as glaucoma (increased pressure within the eyes, which can lead to blindness) and/or seizures, and due to their location, can cause emotional and social issues. All children with hemangiomas or port-wine stains involving the eye should have eye examinations and, if symptoms indicate, brain imaging or further medical evaluation for related complications.

Port-wine stains are often cosmetically treated with cover-up makeup Dermablend or Covermark. Vascular lesion lasers are quite safe and effective in the treatment of port-wine stains and some hemangiomas. Treatment, particularly for facial lesions, should be initiated before school age to minimize teasing in school.

Symptoms

Birthmark Symptoms

Each type of birthmark has its own symptoms. Starting off as a flat red mark, during the first year, the hemangioma soon develops a sponge-like consistency and may grow quite quickly up to two to three inches in diameter. It then stops growing and over time (usually before the fifth birthday) slowly vanishes or begins to disappear. Although the initial redness greatly fades, a child can be left with no markings at all or with permanent, faint discoloration and/or stretched-out skin where the mass of the birthmark involuted. Macular stains are harmless, often require no treatment, and often disappear. Port-wine stains appear at birth, are flat and pink, red, or purplish.

Cause

Birthmark Cause

The exact cause of birthmarks has not been identified.

Treatment

Birthmark Treatment

Most hemangiomas require no treatment, the majority of which resolve themselves by the child's tenth birthday. If the growth encroaches on any orifice (eye, nose, mouth, or genitalia) the lesion should be treated to prevent functional compromise of the orifice. Treatment may also be advised for cosmetic purposes if the birthmark significantly threatens the child's appearance and affects self-esteem. Macular stains don't require treatment.

WHEN TO SEE A DERMATOLOGIST

Consult a dermatologist about any birthmark your child is born with or that develops. They will examine and diagnose the true nature of any discoloration or growth on your child's skin and monitor it during subsequent routine checkups. Like any skin condition, if you observe abnormal changes such as bleeding, bruising, infections, or sudden growth spurts, or changes in marking, coloration, or shape, then consult a physician right away. You should consider cosmetic birthmark treatment before your child reaches school age so they may avoid being teased (and the negative effect cruel comments from other children might have on developing self-esteem and confidence).

Café au Lait Spots

A CAFÉ AU LAIT SPOT, OR CAFÉ AU LAIT MACULE (CALM), mentioned in the section on birthmarks, looks like a pale, coffee-colored stain and can occur anywhere on the body. Other pigmented birthmarks include moles and Mongolian spots. Like many birthmarks, they are not necessarily present at birth but can develop days or weeks later anywhere on the skin and are usually benign.

Café au Lait Symptoms

- Milk coffee in color (light to dark brown)
- Often oval in shape (with smooth or irregular borders)
- Do not fade with age
- Can be three inches in diameter or more

SYMPTOMS

Café au Lait Causes

It's not clear what causes birthmarks. They do seem to occur as a result of an imbalance in the factors that determine the growth and development of skin cells. Some cells get an excess of skin pigment and overgrow. Genetics does not cause a café au lait spot—this is not an inherited issue.

CAUSES

Café au Lait Treatment

In most cases, treatment of café au lait spots is not required. One or two spots on a child's skin is common. However, more than four can be an indication of the presence of another condition such as neurofibromatosis (a hereditary nerve fiber sheath disease, which requires treatment and monitoring). A dermatologist may use pigmented-lesion laser treatment for café au lait spots; however, these treatments often require several sessions, can be painful, and more than 50 percent of the spots tend to recur. In my practice, I generally defer treatment of these lesions until adolescence or early adulthood when the patient can understand the risks and benefits of treating this lesion.

TREATMENT

WHEN TO SEE A DERMATOLOGIST

Monitor café au lait spots for abnormal changes like rapid growth spurts or changes in color or texture. Cosmetic concerns are another reason to seek the expert opinion of a dermatologist, who can recommend treatment options.

Neurofibromatosis

NEUROFIBROMATOSIS (NF1) IS AN INHERITED GENETIC DISORDER that causes tumors to grow on nerve tissue. Also known as von Recklinghausen disease, one symptom of NF1 may be several café au lait spots (at least four to six) on your child's skin. The tumors are frequently benign and the disorder itself is usually mild. However, the effects of the disease can range from hearing impairment to complications of the cardiovascular system and even to cancer. A child who has no birth family history and has café au lait spots should be evaluated for neurofibromatosis.

Neurofibromatosis Symptoms

SYMPTOMS

- Tumors anywhere in the nervous system, including the spinal cord, brain, and the network of nerve cells

- A number of café au lait spots

- Freckles may appear in the child's groin area or in the armpits

- Tumors that grow close to the skin can be felt on the surface as soft bumps

- Tiny tumors may grow on the eye iris (perceptible with special instruments)

- A larger-than-average-sized head

- Issues such as attention deficit hyperactivity disorder (ADHD)

Neurofibromatosis Causes

CAUSES

NF1 is an inherited condition, passed on from the genes of one or both parents. If only one parent carries the gene, the offspring has a 50 percent chance of developing the disorder. It affects boys and girls equally.

TREATMENT

Neurofibromatosis Treatment

In most cases, NF1 tumors are slow-growing and benign. Aside from cosmetic considerations, usually no further treatment is required, although related issues (including ADHD) may require treatment.

WHEN TO SEE A DERMATOLOGIST

NF1 in your child requires professional diagnosis and monitoring.

Sun Damage

SUN DAMAGE IS CAUSED BY CUMULATIVE EXPOSURE to the sun's ultraviolet rays. Chronic sun exposure damages the skin. UVA and UVB rays cause sun damage, aging, and wrinkling (premature aging of the skin). The UVB rays of the sun can burn the skin (causing mutations in the DNA of the skin, which can lead to skin cancer later in life) while the UVA rays can increase the rate of melanoma (though the rays do not burn the skin). A tan is the body's way of attempting to prevent further deeper-level damage to the skin after its DNA has been damaged by UV rays.

Sunburn has far-reaching aftereffects as it is both immediately damaging and can predispose your child to certain types of skin cancer later in life. A suntan is physical evidence of sun damage to the skin and is in no way healthy. Your child's skin needs to be protected at all times and regardless of skin color. The only way to protect your skin from damaging UVA or UVB rays, besides avoiding sun exposure, is through the vigilant use of sun protection. Sunscreen and other products offer UV protection through sun protection factor (SPF).

Sun and SPF

Sunscreen should be applied whenever your child or teen will be in the sun, even for short periods of time. Your child needs sunscreen even if the day is cloudy. Such days can fool us into thinking that we aren't getting sun exposure when in fact we are. The SPF of a product is an indicator of how long the sunscreen can absorb or reflect the sunlight before the rays will affect the skin. A sun screen with zinc oxide or titanium dioxide as an ingredient creates a physical barrier between the skin and the sun. You can cover your child or teen with SPF-rated, tightly woven clothing, hats, and sunglasses.

Sun protection should be applied twenty minutes before sun exposure and reapplied every two hours. Liberally apply sunscreen, using a golf ball-sized dollop (about half an ounce) about twenty to thirty minutes before your child goes out into the sun. Teens, like adults,

A suntan is physical evidence of sun damage to the skin and is in no way healthy.

SPF

can use a whole ounce (about a shot glass-full) of sunscreen. Spending time near water (at the beach or pool) or on ice and snow (ice skating or skiing) increases the chance of sunburn; the sun's rays will be reflected and magnified.

Reapply sunscreen according to the SPF and after swimming or sweating. Use an umbrella, sunshade, or sun tent in the back yard or by the beach or pool. You can be outside and enjoy the fresh air and still avoid the damaging rays of the sun. This is increasingly important if there is any birth family history of skin cancer, particularly melanoma.

Sun Protection and Your Baby

BABIES

If you plan to be in the sun with your baby, try to avoid being out between 10 a.m. and 4 p.m., when the sun burns the brightest. Protect your infant by using a broad-brimmed hat that entirely covers the heat and neck, sunglasses, UV-protective clothing, a UV-protective stroller shade, sun cover, or something else to block the sun. You can use a broad-spectrum sunscreen (one that protects against both UVA and UVB rays) for infants as young as six months of age, but be certain it is a product designed for babies.

Sunscreen and Allergies

SUNSCREEN ALERGIES

Most allergic reactions to sunscreen involve an allergy to para-aminobenzoic acid (PABA) or other chemicals in the sunscreen. Some people are sensitive to PABA. Reactions to PABA include burning or stinging after application or even contact dermatitis (a skin reaction after application) or photoallergic dermatitis (inflammation of the skin after use of the product and exposure to sunlight).

People with chronic skin conditions such as atopic dermatitis are often sensitive to other substances, so caution with chemical sunscreen use is advised. Test sunscreen in a small area on the arm to look for a reaction before applying it to the entire body.

Sun Protection and Teens

TEENS

Your teenager or tween may be unconcerned about excess UV radiation exposure and may even have an interest in purposely tanning in a tanning bed. Some teens, especially girls, like to tan for specific events such as beauty pageants or dances. It is essential for you to explain the risks of sunbathing and tanning. Your teen needs to know that tanned skin is damaged skin. Your child needs to know that naturally darker skin does not protect against skin cancer and that people who tan indoors are 74 percent more likely to get melanoma than those people who have never tanned indoors.[4]

More than 1,500 people die from cancer daily[5], including one person dying from malignant melanoma each hour.[6] There are different kinds of skin cancer and some are more treatable than others or have a better prognosis if caught early.

Asian American and African American melanoma patients are more likely than Caucasians to be diagnosed with an advanced stage of melanoma.

Your teenager needs to know about UVA and UVB rays and how UVA rays penetrate more deeply into the skin (all the way to the dermis) where they can damage the immune system and cause melanoma. Teach your teen that melanoma is a serious and deadly type of skin cancer. Did you know that Asian American and African American melanoma patients are more likely than Caucasians to be diagnosed with an advanced stage of the disease?[7] Melanoma is far less common than basal cell carcinoma and other skin cancers yet far more deadly.[8] The later melanoma is diagnosed, the more likely the cancer has metastasized or spread and the harder it is to treat.

Some teens are passionate about athletics and may play sports or participate in other activities outside in the sun during the heat of the day. Your teenager needs to know that daily sunscreen application is required and nonnegotiable. Other teens may feel under pressure to be cool and look a certain way. Hollywood actors and other celebrities, whom teens may wish to emulate, are often depicted as tan.

4 Lazovich D, Vogel RI, Berwick M, Weinstock MA, Anderson KE, Warshaw EM. Indoor tanning and risk of melanoma: a case-control study in a highly-exposed population. *Cancer Epidem Biomar Prev* 2010 June; 19(6):1557-1568.

5 American Cancer Society. 2010 Cancer Facts and Figures. (http://cancer.org/Research/CancerFactsFigures/CancerFactsFigures/cancer-facts-and-figures-2010)

6 American Cancer Society. Cancer Facts & Figures 2010. http://cancer.org/research/cancerfactsfigures/cancerfactsfigures/cancer-facts-and-figures-2010 . Accessed July 1, 2011.

7 Cress RD, Holly EA. Incidence of cutaneous melanoma among non-Hispanic whites, Hispanics, Asians, and blacks: an analysis of California cancer registry data, 1988-93. *Cancer Causes Control* 1997; 8:246-52.

8 The Burden of Skin Cancer. National Center for Chronic Disease Prevention and Health Promotion. http://.cdc.gov/HealthyYouth/skincancer/facts.htm. Accessed July 1, 2011.

Tanning salons may promote their services by exaggerating the benefits of exposure to UV rays and suggesting that tanning, or increased melanin production, is natural and healthful. It is up to you to educate and protect your child. I often tell my patients, "If you were meant to be brown, you would have been born that way. Be who you are."

Allow your teenager to shop for his or her own 100-percent UV-protective sunglasses and a hat that provides sun protection. Teenage boys and girls both can wear specially manufactured 100-percent UV-sun-protective clothing. Teen girls can wear loose-fitting cover ups, including beautiful sarongs, along with broad-brimmed hats, scarves, and eyewear. Keep a sun protection kit in the car, along with an attractive sun umbrella and extra hats, scarves, and 100-percent UV-protective sunglasses. Even a single incident of childhood sunburn, or use of an indoor tanning bed, dramatically increases your child's chance of skin cancer in the future.

Sunburn

IF YOUR BABY, CHILD, OR TEEN GETS SUNBURNED, treat it as a serious condition. For an infant or very young child, it could be considered a medical emergency. All babies, whatever their skin tones, have especially sensitive skin. Melanin production isn't fully developed in babies, so their skin is vulnerable to sunlight. If your child gets sunburned, get him or her out of the sun immediately. Sunburn is skin damage. The following symptoms are serious:

Extreme Sunburn Symptoms

- Pain
- Blistering of the skin
- Inflammation/reddening of the skin
- Decreased urine output
- Fever/a temperature over 100°
- Chills
- Lethargy/fatigue

SYMPTOMS

There is no immediate cure for sunburn, but there are things you can do to help the situation. Give your child age-appropriate fluids to help rehydrate him or her. Apply cool compresses and a moisturizer to the child's skin. Try keeping the moisturizer in the refrigerator so it will be more comforting. Avoid products containing alcohol as it is drying. Aspirin has been linked to Reye's syndrome, which is rare but potentially fatal, so do not give it to your child.

If your child has severe sunburn along with a headache, confusion, fainting, nausea, or vomiting, take him or her to an emergency room. Consult your physician before using over-the-counter sunburn products (some have been linked to serious conditions, especially in toddlers). Your dermatologist or a physician can prescribe the best treatment for a child's severe sunburn. In cases of extreme sunburn, a child may have to be admitted to the hospital, require strong prescription pain-relieving and anti-inflammatory medication, and IV fluids for rehydrating.

As the skin heals itself, continue to use the treatment recommended by your doctor. Avoid popping or breaking any blisters. Once blisters have been disrupted, risk of infection increases. The skin will begin to peel after several days. Continue to apply moisturizer several times a day to the peeling areas. The best remedy for sunburn is to avoid it. You'll learn how to make a sun protection kit for your child in the next section.

Sun Protection Kit

TO EDUCATE AND PROTECT YOUR CHILD from the UV rays of the sun, make a sun protection kit. Be certain to thoroughly explain the purpose and use of the sun protection kit. Take the time to focus on and enjoy this project with your child to make it a positive teaching experience and a time to bond and connect more deeply.

Let your child or teen help you assemble the sun protection kit. Allow them to choose their sunglasses and a broad-brimmed hat. You will need a small to medium-sized decorated box or zippered bag. If possible, have your child or teen decorate the box or bag. This will give them a sense of pride and ownership, and they will be more invested in using the kit. Keep the kit handy in the car.

The following is a list of what you need for your child's sun protection kit:

- Hat: wide-brimmed with back flap to cover the back of the neck if possible

- Sunscreen: water resistant, broad spectrum (UVA/UVB protective), with a minimum SPF of 30

- Sunglasses (designed for your child's age with 100-percent UVA/UVB protection)

- UV Protective Clothing (or regular clothing that covers the body entirely)

- SPF Lip Balm

Remember to apply and reapply sunscreen according to the instructions, usually within a couple hours of the each application. If your child is active and sweaty or has been in the water, you will need to reapply sunscreen more often.

SUN PROTECTION KIT

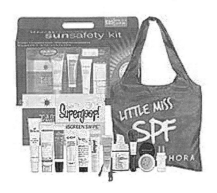

Pediatric Skin Cancer

SKIN CANCER IS ABNORMAL SKIN CELL GROWTH. The primary cause of all skin cancers is DNA mutation of skin cells after exposure to UV radiation from the sun, tanning beds, and tanning lamps. Although there is a much lower incidence of cancer, including skin cancer, in children compared to adults, children do get skin cancer. Pediatric skin cancer affects children of any skin color.

The three types of skin cancer are named for the layer of skin cell where they originate: squamous cell skin cancer (in squamous skin cells), basal cell skin cancer (in basal skin cells), and the deadly melanoma (in melanocytes). Skin phototype, strength of the immune system, and exposure to UVA and UVB radiation (whether from the sun or tanning beds or booths) increase the chance of developing squamous cell or basal cell skin cancers, which are the two most common types of skin cancer.[9] Skin cancer patients have a good prognosis if the cancer is diagnosed and treated early.

Squamous Cell and Basal Cell Skin Cancer Symptoms

SYMPTOMS

- A sore that doesn't heal
- Skin areas that are small, raised, shiny, and waxy
- Skin areas that are raised and red or reddish-brown
- Skin that is scaly, bleeds, and is crusty
- Skin that looks like firm scar tissue
- Flat, rough, red or brown, scaly skin tissue

9 American Cancer Society, 2011. Skin Cancer Prevention and Early Detection, accessed 1 July 2011, <http://www.cancer.org/acs/groups/cid/documents/webcontent/003184-pdf.pdf>

A dermatologist can examine the skin to diagnose squamous cell or basal cell skin cancer and may examine the lymph nodes as well. A biopsy, or skin sample, may be performed. The biopsy will then be sent to a dermatopathologist (a pathologist specializing in skin disease). If a growth is found to be precancerous, your doctor may recommend monitoring, more testing, or surgery. If squamous cell or basal cell cancer is found, the tumor may be surgically removed and more tests may be conducted to determine if the cancer has spread. Chemotherapy or radiation may be required.

About 500 children are diagnosed with pediatric melanoma annually in the US, and 90 percent of those cases occur in girls aged 10 to19.[10] About 65 percent of melanoma can be attributed to UVA and UVB radiation from exposure to sunlight,[11] so minimizing exposure to sunlight (and preventing sunburn) will reduce the likelihood that your child will get melanoma. Unfortunately, incidence of childhood melanoma is increasing, though generally the prognosis is good: large-scale studies report a 74 percent to 80 percent survival rate after five years with local excision (except in metastatic or regional disease or advanced cases).[12] As treatable as early-diagnosed childhood melanoma is, any increased risk of childhood melanoma is too great. Ideally, you will not allow your child to participate in high-risk skin behaviors, such as sunbathing and tanning or spending time in the sun, without appropriate sun protection.

Research indicates that childhood melanoma is very similar to melanoma in young adults except that there are more cases in males and some of the cancer sites are atypical.[13]

---

10 Strous JJ, Fears TR, Tucker MA, Wayne AS. Pediatric melanoma: risk factor and survival analysis of the surveillance, epidemiology and end results database. J Clin Oncol 2005; 23:4735-41.

11 Armstrong BK, Kricker A. How much melanoma is caused by sun exposure? Mel Res 1993 December 3(6):395-401.

12 Strouse JJ, Fears TR, Tucher MA, Wayne AS. Pediatric melanoma: risk factor and survival analysis of the surveillance, epidemiology and end results database. J Clin Oncol. 2005; 23(21):4735-4741.

13 Strouse JJ, Fears TR, Tucher MA, Wayne AS. Pediatric melanoma: risk factor and survival analysis of the surveillance, epidemiology and end results database. J Clin Oncol. 2005; 23(21):4735-4741.

Melanoma Skin Cancer Symptoms

- A change in the size, shape, or color or a mole (ABCDE[14])

- A mole that has irregular borders (edges) or is asymmetrical

- A mole or growth that appears (where there wasn't one before)

- A new mole

- A mole that is more than one color

- A mole that itches or is sore

- A mole that oozes, bleeds, or ulcerates (opens like a sore/wound)

- A new growth that grows quickly, bleeds, or has multiple colors

Factors that increase the risk of skin cancer include:

- Having fair or light skin tone (blondes or redheads with light eyes, who freckle and sunburn easily, are less protected from the sun's UV rays).

- Heavy sun exposure.

- A history of sunburns. Sunburn is skin damage and increases the likelihood of cellular mutation from the radiation.

- A great many moles or an abnormal mole.

- Being at-risk genetically or having one or more siblings or parents diagnosed with skin cancer.

- Having had skin cancer before.

- An immune system that is weakened or struggling from dealing with another disease.

- Drinking alcohol or smoking.

- Exposure to known carcinogens; arsenic is a toxin known to cause skin cancer[15] and is often found in well water.

- Living in a certain locality (such as Australia, which has the highest rate of skin cancer in the world).

---

14 Remember ABCDE? (A—Asymmetry, B—Borders (irregular), C—Color (more than one), D—Diameter (bigger than 6mm) and E—Evolving (changing or NEW moles).

15 Smith, A.H et al., 1992, 'Cancer risks from arsenic in drinking water', Environmental Health Perspectives, 97:259–267.

You can reduce the risk of skin cancer by:

- Minimizing your child's exposure to sunlight (UVA and UVB radiation).

- Promoting activities in the shade.

- Providing sunscreen and UV-protective clothing and headgear.

- Monitoring your child's skin, being certain to note and regularly check moles, freckles, skin tags, or other growths, and watching for changes.

- Taking your child for a dermatologic consult if you notice any skin changes.

- Being certain your baby, child, or teen has regular well-baby and well-child medical evaluations (your pediatrician may catch a change before you do).

- Preventing sunburn (avoid tanning bed and unnecessary sunlight exposure).

You cannot control genetics (and you may not know the genetic history of your adopted child), yet you can lay the foundation for a lifetime of healthy skin by protecting then teaching your child the importance of sun protection.

PATIENT STORY

I recently had an adoptive family come in for skin evaluation. The parents were Caucasian and the child was from Guatemala. Both parents had significant sun damage and sunburns on the day of the visit. Their child also was very tan. When I asked if their child wore sun protection, they responded that she didn't need it because she had such naturally dark skin. We talked about proper sun protection for her, and I shared with them the fact that Bob Marley died of a melanoma; skin cancer can and does occur in darker skin.

Part II: The Hair and Scalp

About Hair

Human hair is made of a type of protein called keratin.

HAIR OFFERS SOME PROTECTION from the rays of the sun, provides some warmth in colder climates and cooling in hotter climates, and when styled, is considered a fashion accessory. Hair can affect our self-image and self-esteem, as it has social and cultural significance.

Some babies are born with hair and others are born with so little they are considered bald. Human hair is made of a type of protein called keratin (the same material that our fingernails and toenails are made of). Hair grows out of hair follicles in the dermis of the skin and scalp. Each human hair has two parts: a soft, thick hair bulb, or root, and the upper part, or hair shaft.

What you eat and drink directly affects the health of your hair. Eating a healthy diet that includes pure water, fresh fruits and vegetables, protein, and fiber will help your blood supply important nutrients and chemical compounds to the hair roots. Other things affect our hair, including genetic or inherited issues. Like other human characteristics and features, there are variations in hair, including density, thickness, color, and texture.

Hair texture, color, and thickness vary widely even within ethnic groups. Each child's hair texture will ultimately depend on his or her genetic makeup. Hair texture, like skin color, may cross perceived common ethnic boundaries. In some cases, black or very dark-skinned children may naturally have straight hair. In another case, a child with light skin may be born with extremely kinky hair. The hair of Asian children is generally very straight and dark in color.

Every child has an individualized hair texture and color. All hair is beautiful. No hair is "bad" or "good." It is up to you to teach your child to avoid negative terminology and be culturally sensitive to themselves and others. Whether a child's hair is kinky, curly, wavy, straight, thick, medium, or fine, he or she can maintain and love his or her hair, and feel attractive and loved.

Hair Types

HAIR IS IMPORTANT TO PEOPLE. Our hair, like our facial shape, is part of what makes us both unique and attractive. One of the joys of caring for children is grooming them, including caring for and styling their hair. It is very common for adoptive parents to wonder what their baby or child will look like as he/she gets older.

The answer to this question is in your child's genes. Most likely the baby or child will display hair traits similar to the birth mother or father. As an adoptive parent, you may not have information about the birth parents. Hair is mostly "what you see is what you get," but that isn't always the case with babies. Some babies are bald at birth. Other infants have heads of thick, wavy hair. Another baby may have straight, fine hair that is thin or grows in patches. But the hair a child is born with may not be the hair he or she ends up with. Newborn hair is baby hair. Baby hair typically falls out, then new hair grows. No matter what kind of hair color, texture, or thickness your children have, you should appreciate their hair and make sure they know it.

Hair follicle shape determines hair texture.

- Round follicles result in straight hair.

- Oval follicles result in wavy hair.

- Flat follicles result in curly hair.

- A flat, spiraled follicle will result in tightly coiled hair.

You will want to learn techniques, and the best tools and products, to style your adopted child's hair. Your child may have a different ethnic background. They may have hair that is entirely different from your hair or any hair that you have ever worked with or styled. The next section has frequently asked questions about hair. Following that are sections on hair-care basics and how to assemble a hair-care kit for your child. An important section after that covers most common hair issues you will deal with while taking care of your child.

The hair a child is born with may not be the hair he or she ends up with.

Remember to avoid using negative words to describe your child's hair. Saying "Red hair just isn't attractive," "I don't know what we're going to do with your hair," "Your hair is impossible," "You're hair is nappy," or "I hate your hair," is unkind and will only upset your child. Everything of value takes time and effort, including creating and maintaining healthy or beautiful hair and a nice-looking style. Show your child how special he or she is and how beautiful. Teach your child that his or her lovely hair requires care, time, and effort. Make "doing hair care" a special time with your children. This time is an opportunity to love and nurture them while teaching them lifelong self-care skills. You can listen to music and be close to them. This special bonding time simultaneously allows you to gently and lovingly care for their hair, or teach them to do so, while at the same time reinforcing proper loving self-care.

Self-esteem is an important foundation for personal and professional success in life. Parental attitudes affect children's attitudes toward themselves and others. Make sure your children learn to appreciate and nurture themselves and their particular type of beauty or good looks. Every person, every type of face, hair, and body are unique.

Try to avoid doing your child's hair when you are in a hurry; this can be stressful and create drama as well as physical pain as you may end up tugging and hurting the scalp. Also, when you rush while doing hair styling, it can easily turn out to be "a bad hair day" for your child. It may be difficult to always find time to properly style your child's hair. If you don't have much time, try using a headband or other hair accessory, such as a scarf or hat.

Self-esteem is an important foundation for personal and professional success in life.

Hair FAQs

CERTAIN QUESTIONS ABOUT HAIR AND SCALP care for children come up more frequently than others. A professional stylist who is experienced in caring for and styling hair like your child's is a good resource. Some frequently asked questions are:

1. How can I learn to take care of my adopted child's hair?

Study and research your children's hair type and learn methods of care and styling so you'll become skilled in caring for their hair (and teach them to do the same). The internet is an amazing resource with blogs and websites (some with videos and ebooks) offering specific instruction in hair care and styling methods.

2. How fast does hair grow?

Hair grows at different rates. However, in general, you can expect it to grow from a quarter of an inch to a half inch per month. Curly hair, because it is coiled, appears to grow more slowly. Hair length is determined in part by the length of the growth cycle, which varies among individuals and even between hair located in different parts of the same person's body. This explains why the hair of one's eyebrows will grow to only a certain length and the hair on the head of the same person will grow much longer—the growth cycle varies.

3. Is a brush or comb better for my child's hair?

Either a brush or comb is appropriate for your child's hair. Wide-toothed combs can be great for parting and detangling hair, while brushes are good for gently brushing hair. Some people feel that a boar bristle brush or a wooden rake comb are the very best hair-care tools. What is important is that you learn to use all hair-care tools properly before you style your child's hair—and remember to be gentle. Many scalp and hair issues can be avoided if you avoid tugging a child's hair and pulling the hair too tightly. Proper brushing, combing, and detangling techniques are essential.

4. How often do I need to shampoo my child's hair?

This depends on the texture of the hair. Generally, the curlier the hair, the less often you need to wash it. Straight hair should be washed every one to three days whereas very curly or kinky hair can be washed every ten to fourteen days. Be careful not to shampoo your child's hair too often. Shampooing too often is damaging to hair, but more so for curly hair. Do not shampoo curly or kinky hair every day, as it will strip much of the moisture from your child's hair.

5. What kind of hair products should my child use?

Your child needs hair products that are ideal for his or her hair type and, preferably, do not have synthetic or harsh chemicals or irritants. You should use products that are designed for that hair type. Hair is keratin (dead protein) and needs to be moisturized but not made oily. Different products work for different hair; experiment with your child's hair and try a variety of hair products.

SHAMPOO

Hair Products—Shampoos

Shampoo is designed to remove dirt and excess oil (sebum) from dirty hair. The right shampoo can radically affect the appearance and health of hair. Many shampoo commercials promise that the product can restore, nurture, nourish, or "feed" hair. Many of these claims are not entirely honest. Ideally a shampoo will clean the hair without entirely stripping out precious natural oils. You may need to wash your child's hair less often than you think. Hair is not unlike fabric. Washing the same shirt every day will wear out the fabric sooner.

Wet Shampoo—

This type of shampoo generally offers options for specific hair types (such as baby, color-treated, damaged, or dandruff-ridden hair). Some wet shampoos are more moisturizing than others, so be certain to read the ingredients. Use a tearless baby shampoo for infants and young children (although some older children and adults use baby shampoo, as it is very gentle).

Wet Shampoo/Conditioner (all-in-one product)—

These combination products may work fine for average, healthy hair types and textures. However, a shampoo/conditioner product may be *too* moisturizing for oily hair and *not* moisturizing enough for very dry hair. Be wary of products that are supposedly great for all hair types.

Dry Shampoo—

May be useful when traveling or camping or when you otherwise don't have the time or facilities to easily use wet shampoo.. Your teen may like to use dry shampoo after workouts, to avoid overuse of wet shampoos. Keep in mind that dry shampoo isn't ideal for all hair types and doesn't clean hair so much as absorb oil. Some dry shampoos may leave a white residue or powder (although others are color-matched), so you may need to experiment to find one that works for you and your child. Also, be certain to read the ingredients label and decide whether or not you are comfortable using those ingredients on your child's hair. A great thing about dry shampoos is that you avoid the need to use water and heat (dryers or flattening irons) afterward.

Hair Products—Conditioners

CONDITIONER

Conditioners are designed to condition, or moisturize, the hair. Carefully choosing a conditioner can add shine to and protect hair and, like a good shampoo, can drastically affect hair's appearance and health.

Moisturizers—

These conditioners have more compounds that are similar to the natural sebaceous oils in the scalp and also for retaining moisture than other types of conditioners. Most children need to use a moisturizer whenever their hair is washed.

Reconstructors—

This type of conditioner can help eliminate frizz and is designed for processed or chemically damaged or heat-damaged hair. If often has ingredients such as protein in it; this allows the product to strengthen, moisturize, and more intensely condition the hair.

Acidifiers—

These are conditioners with a pH below 3.5, which is good to compact, or close, the cuticle of the hair. This seals in moisture and generally will create bouncy, shiny hair and is good for hair that gets knotty and/or tangled. Detanglers often fall into this category.

Kinky, curly, or dry hair needs moisture and oil but not grease. Oils—natural or added through conditioner—don't travel as easily down a curly hair shaft, so it is important to use a creamier moisturizing shampoo for coarse, curly, kinky, or wavy hair. It is important to use a small amount and gently apply it to your child's hair each time you have shampooed. Be attentive to the hair ends, placing most of the conditioner at the tips to help lessen dryness and nurture any split ends.

6. Why is my child losing hair and what can I do about it?

A child's hair and scalp are sensitive, and hair loss is not uncommon. An infant or child may experience hair loss due to friction from overuse of hair accessories, too-tight hairstyles, or because of a disease or condition. Hair conditions that cause hair loss in children include a fungal infection called tinea capitis, or alopecia areata (thought to be caused by immune system dysfunction), hair traction trauma (too-tight hair accessories or friction of some kind or chemical burns), trichotillomania (a nervous habit of pulling at or pulling out the hair), or telogen effluvium (a problem in the natural hair growth cycle), among others. There are other issues, including serious medical conditions and eating disorders, which can cause or contribute to hair loss. Hair loss issues need a correct diagnosis to determine the best treatment. See a dermatologist and follow his or her recommendation to resolve pediatric hair-loss issues.

7. My child has a lot of hair and doesn't like it when I comb or brush it. How can I get her to sit still while I do her hair?

When styling hair, be certain you have your child's comb and other tools handy on a little table or shelf. Put on a special movie or music to occupy your child's attention while you do his or her hair. Make the experience special. Whatever you provide for her to focus on, only use it while you are coming or brushing her hair. If your child needs a break from brushing or coming, then turn the music or movie off until she is ready to sit down and let you continue. You could also have a toy, soft blanket, or stuffed animal for her to hold (a special hair buddy). Have a healthful drink or snack handy. Hair-care time is easier for everyone if you create a pleasant, gentle experience of loving connection.

8. At what age can my child go to a hair salon?

A baby's hair can be cut or trimmed whenever it is long, but it is safest if you cut or trim hair at home, perhaps while your child is sleeping or calm, until the child is at least one year old. When a child reaches this age, he or she has the muscle control to hold up his or her head and sit up in a chair safely, without slumping. He or she is also less likely to be afraid of the experience. Your child will likely be happiest in a salon designed for children that offers television, specially designed chairs, and other child-friendly items. Try to adapt to your child's needs if he or she is uncomfortable around strangers or in a new environment. Keep in mind that blow dryers can be very scary for toddlers and young children.

9. Will my son go bald from wearing a hat or baseball cap all the time?

Baldness is a genetic trait passed from both the paternal and maternal family lines. But hats or other hair accessories (including headbands and tight caps) that rub the head or pull the hair and cause friction *can* cause hair loss. A cap that is loose, not tight, and doesn't pull or rub hair should not be a problem.

10. My child pulls his sibling's hair. Should I pull his hair to show him how it feels, so he'll stop?

Children learn best by example, so, no, it's not a good idea to show your child what not to do by doing it. Find out why your child is pulling the other child's hair. Your child may need to learn new, healthy ways to express anger. Sometimes children pull hair because they like the way it feels. If your baby or child seems to like pulling hair, gently explain that it hurts the other person and offer an alternative tactile experience (such as playing with clay or Play-Doh) or patting a special stuffed animal. Speak with your pediatrician if your child pulls hair regularly; hair-pulling can become a compulsive pattern of behavior and should be brought under control.

<u>Getting Started: Basic Hair Care</u>

BE ESPECIALLY GENTLE WITH A BABY'S HEAD and hair. In order to allow room for the brain to grow, a baby's skull plate is not fully fused at birth. The areas where the bone is not yet fused at the top of the head are called soft spots, or fontanels. Even when the fontanels disappear, you need to be very careful, as your child's hair follicles are not fully developed. Your baby's hair and scalp need extremely gentle care.

General tips and warnings for styling your little one's hair:

TIPS

- Never pull the hair too tightly or try to force styles that can't be accomplished.

- Be wary of using rubber bands or hair ornaments that could easily come out of your baby's or toddler's hair and find their way into her mouth. These are choking hazards!

- Be aware of the weather. Protect your baby's sensitive hair and tiny head from the elements (sun, heat, and cold).

- Shampoo once every week, or every two weeks if he or she has a very dry scalp. Use a gentle baby shampoo specifically made for your child's hair type. Do not shampoo daily.

- If your child's hair or scalp gets dirty on a non-shampoo day, you can rub the scalp and hair clean with a wet washcloth or a dry shampoo.

- Use a little soft bristle baby brush to gently tidy the hair.

- Brush a baby's or child's hair in the direction of his or her natural hair pattern. Newborn hair requires little maintenance.

After a few months, a baby's hair texture will change. Some babies have lots of hair at birth or a few months later. Other babies are bald, and their hair shows no signs of growth. If your child's hair grows very slowly, don't worry. Nothing is wrong. It can take from one to three years for some babies to grow a full head of hair. Their hair may never be thick, if their natural texture is thin and fine. Be patient. Don't attempt to force your baby's or child's hair to do what you want it to do. Allow the hair to grow in naturally.

Hair loss is natural for an infant. Your baby's hair may fall out entirely or one side of the head. Either way it's completely normal. Hormonal changes often cause hair loss; immediately following birth, a baby undergoes hormonal changes that often lead to hair loss. If you notice that your child is only losing hair on the sides, it may be due to an equally harmless reason. The neck muscles of babies develop slowly, so they often rub their heads against objects, like crib mattresses. This causes them to lose hair along the sides and back of the head. But don't worry; your baby's hair will grow in, all over, at some point.

Immediately following birth, a baby undergoes hormonal changes that often lead to hair loss.

Hair Care Steps

Hair care starts with a clean hair. This section offers detailed, step-by-step instructions for washing your child's hair. Before washing your child's hair, carefully and gently brush it (your child's particular hair texture will dictate which type of hair brush or comb is best). Then shampoo and condition your child's hair. Use warm, not hot, water to minimize hair damage and breakage. Once your child's hair is clean (you may have to experiment with shampoos and conditioners to find the products that are ideal for your child), condition it to seal in moisture and make his or her hair even more beautiful.

Washing and Conditioning

1) Massage a quarter-sized amount of tear-free shampoo, with warm or tepid water, into your child's hair.

2) Rinse the hair with cool water.

3) Apply a basic conditioner (to the ends only, if your child has oily hair) and a more moisturizing conditioner, specific to your child's hair type and texture, if your child tends to have dry hair.

4) Gently comb through the hair with a wide-tooth comb while conditioner is still in the hair to help detangle.

5) Carefully rinse the hair with cool water (again being careful not to tangle, snarl, or knot the ends). If your child isn't too uncomfortable with the temperature, use cold water for the final rinse.

6) Blot the hair with a towel (ideally a special absorptive towel just for this purpose).

7) Style your child's hair when it is dry, or while it is damp or wet, depending upon the hair type and texture.

Whatever your child's natural hair type and texture, research the styles that will suit him or her best. Their hair will be easier to care for and maintain if it is styled. Keep in mind that face shape, as well as hair texture and type, affects what style would best suit your child. The great news is that your child's hair, in the absence of a scalp or hair condition, should grow fast. You can experiment with several hairstyles and cuts to see which one suits your child at his or her age, given face shape, hair type and texture, and your lifestyle and the amount of time you can reasonably spend on maintaining the hair. Every style starts with a clean head of hair.

Below you'll find information about hair textures and types and step-by-step instructions in how to create certain basic hair styles for your child.

Hair Textures and Types

Each type of hair should be styled in whatever way is ideal for its type. The following information should be useful to you, but this book is not dedicated to hair or hair styling. Look for books or online information to guide you in choosing a cut and style that is ideal for your child.

Straight Hair Basics

STRAIGHT HAIR

Caring for straight hair is a little different than caring for other hair. Straight hair may be fine, medium, or coarse, or a combination of these three textures. In very straight hair, keratin bundles in the hair also tend to be straight. This means the hair shaft is thicker and almost completely round and so, more than any other type, straight hair is often considered easier to manage and maintain, especially when it is shiny and in terrific condition. Straight hair does have a tendency to fall flat, but when styled according to type, it can be maintained without too much effort.

Straight Hair Styles

When cutting straight hair, you may prefer to choose a fuss-free, simple style that requires little maintenance. Straight hair can be cut with a blunt end or graduated into layers. Layers will give hair more texture and may make the hair appear to have more volume. You could try a shoulder-length style with layers for your child. This style will help to frame the face. For children with straight hair, the layered look helps them naturally keep their style, without the use of a lot of hair products.

Straight hair can be braided or put into ponytails or pigtails or similar styles. Straight hair looks great clean and brushed and held back with a headband. Straight hair may not hold a wave or curl very well, but if you use hot rollers or a curling iron, it can be a great look as well. Depending upon your child's face shape, a style such as a bob or pageboy may look especially nice if they have straight or nearly straight hair.

Curly, Kinky, and Wavy Hair Basics

Scientists do not fully understand why hair grows straight or curly or wavy, although they know it is partly determined by genetics and other factors, including follicle shape. Some curly-headed children may have straight hair later in life, and vice versa. The longer the hair grows, the more accentuated the natural character of the hair becomes.

All hair twists as it grows. The number of twists in a given length of hair determines how curly it is. The more twists in a hair shaft, the curlier the hair. The hair of people with really kinky hair twists much more frequently than other hair. Some hair, for instance, can have up to twelve times as many twists per centimeter than other hair.

Kinky hair shafts are more oval in shape and have more distinct edges. The cuticle is kinked at the edges and more easily damaged, or prone to breakage, at these points. This particular shape exposes kinky hair to differing forms of physical and chemical trauma. This means that both kinky and curly hair need extra care in handling and conditioning. Combing or brushing kinky hair excessively could damage it.

Curly, Kinky, and Wavy Hair Styles

Curly, kinky, and wavy hair isn't "bad" or "worse than" other hair. It is what it is. It requires certain styling, cutting, and care. The way you treat your children and their hair will teach them to love themselves and their physical features (including their hair). When cutting curly, kinky, or wavy hair, scissors and a dry or slightly damp cut are preferred. Use of a razor on many hair types can be damaging. With a child who has curly, kinky, or wavy hair, you may find that you prefer an easy, simple hairstyle that requires low maintenance. This generally means natural hair.

"Natural hair" means that you will wash the hair, moisturize it, and use appropriate products so it can air dry into soft, no-frizz waves or curls. No matter how gentle you are, styling puts tension on the hair, which may result in breakage and damage. Curly, wavy, or kinky hair can be can be styled naturally or carefully put into a particular hairstyle.

Curly, wavy, or kinky hair can generally hold a hairstyle much better than straight hair. Like straight hair, curly, wavy, or kinky hair can be braided, put into cornrows, ponytails, pigtails, or similar styles. Beware of harsh chemicals, inexpert stylists, and hot styling tools. Overuse of a flat iron or curling iron can seriously damage your child's beautiful curly, wavy, or kinky hair. Many hair salons will provide a product or styling consultation. There are many blogs, especially for parents of children with textured hair. Depending upon your child's face shape, you may prefer a definite cut and style. Be certain the hairstylist understands your child's hair type and texture. Some really attractive hairstyles for kinky hair include Bantu twists, double-stranded twists, or puffs. The following pages include how-to information for simple and basic styles.

Double-Stranded Twists

Hair that has been styled into double-stranded twists can be shampooed without unraveling the twists. If the style flattens during sleep, lightly spritz your child's hair with a spray bottle containing a mix of water and moisturizing oil such as argan.

TWISTS

Needed Items:

- Comb (may also need a wide-tooth comb for detangling hair)
- Hair clips to secure the strands
- Tiny rubber bands (preferably cloth covered), if necessary
- Hair oil and gel, depending on type of hair
- Plastic spray bottle

Instructions:

1. Decide the size you want the twists to be.
2. Using a comb, part off a section of hair in a half-inch square.
3. Clip the rest of the hair out of your way.
4. Comb out the parted-off section. Apply some oil, or an appropriate moisturizing product, if the hair is dry. If some curls are loose and won't stay together when twisted, apply some gel on the section to hold that hair in place.

5. Use both of your hands to separate the parted-off section into two.

6. Cross one hand over the other, to cross the sections of hair. Switch hands.

7. Repeat so that the hair twists together like a rope. The curls should wrap around themselves and hold the double twists in. If the twists come out, secure them with a tiny rubber band.

8. Repeat these steps until all the hair is twisted.

Tip: Twist the hair in the direction you want the twist to lie.

Simple Braids

Braids are a quick, easy, adorable hairstyle for playtime or school.

Needed Items:

- Comb (both a rattail as well as a wide-tooth comb for detangling hair)
- Rubber bands (preferably cloth-covered)

Instructions:

1. Pull your child's hair into a ponytail.

2. Section off the hair into three equal sections. Take two sections of the hair in one hand and take the third section of hair in the other hand.

3. Cross the third section into the middle of the first two sections of hair and continue to criss-cross sections, switching them from your right to left hand. Keep the sections fairly tight so that the braid is not so loose it will fall out.

4. Continue until there is no more hair left to braid. Place a coated elastic band on the end to secure the braid.

BRAIDS

Puffs

Puffs are a simple and relatively easy style, although you may have to practice a bit to feel very happy with your efforts. Puffs may not last as long as braids or other styles, but they are usually fairly quick to do and don't put excessive tension on the scalp.

Needed Items:

- A soft brush or comb
- One or more bobby pins
- Hair spray, gel and/or moisturizer

Instructions:

1. Wash and condition hair making sure it is free of tangles and knots. If necessary, apply product to smooth out the hair and to help it stay in place.
2. Separate the section of hair you want for the puff.
3. Twist the selected section of hair until you reach the scalp.
4. Pull the twisted hair forward to create the puff. Secure the twisted hair with one or more bobby pins.
5. Repeat these steps until many sections of hair or "puffs" are surrounding your child's face.

There are numerous attractive and simple ways to create hairstyles that you may like to try on your child. Your teen may have very specific ideas about what he or she prefers; if possible, allow your children to choose their own hairstyles. Choosing a hairstyle, like choosing clothing, is a very personal form of self-expression, and your child will naturally want to make his or her own choices.

You may have your own ideas about what is appropriate, but it is important for your child to have a voice in life and make choices. Your children can be empowered and learn about choices and consequences if you let them make as many choices as possible.

Adornments: Barrettes, Clips, Headbands, Scarves, and Head Wraps

Hair accessories come in many different shapes and sizes. As well as preventing damage and securing your child's hair style, they are adornments or decorations. Some hair accessories such as caps protect your child's hairstyle while he or she plays, naps, or sleeps. A sleep cap can help prevent the frizzies (when shorter wiry/kinky hairs manage to escape the style) and extend the life of a hairstyle. Caps and scarves are great ways to create an instant style without much time or effort. These can be great if your child's hair is not styled and you have to make an unplanned excursion.

Barrettes

Barrettes are used for gathering, fastening, or clipping the hair. They come in all sizes. Some are more functional; others are especially pretty. Barrettes are suitable for most hair lengths. There are even tiny Velcro-closure barrettes for infants. Make sure that the barrette you choose is appropriate for the weight of your child's hair. Be sure the barrettes aren't too tight. Barrettes can be placed in the hair in subtle and invisible ways to accentuate the child's hairstyle.

Jaw Clip

As an alternative to a hair tie, a jaw clip can keep long hair up and out of the way. Jaw clips come in a variety of sizes, colors, and patterns and are usually chosen for more casual occasions and to keep hair away from the face when washing or showering. Mini jaw clips are child favorites as they can give the hair a cool, "piecey" look that some kids love.

Snap Clip

Another child's favorite is the snap clip. It makes a snapping sound when it is closed. Easy to use, they come in a range of sizes and colors and give a more secure hold than the jaw clip. Securing pieces of hair of any type and texture, they are ideal for keeping hair in place during playtime and sports.

Headbands

Headbands come in many different shapes and sizes and they are always in fashion. Unlike scarves, headbands are not wrapped around the head but should be chosen for the correct size for the child's head. If it's too small, it could hurt and cut off vital blood circulation to the scalp. Like any headgear, a too-tight headband can rub and cause hair breakage or loss. Be certain that all headgear fits your child's head.

Headbands work with all hairstyles—long or short, curly or straight—and are very useful for keeping hair back away from the face and out of the eyes. **Avoid using headbands with metal or plastic teeth in curly or kinky hair, as these can cause breakage.**

Scarves and Head Wraps

Unlike headbands that stretch around the head, scarves are wrapped or tied around the head. Variations abound depending on the type, width, length of fabric, and the number of times it is wrapped around the head. As well as being stylish, scarves can preserve a hairstyle and shield your child's head and scalp from the wind and sun.

Avoiding Future Problems with Hair

The overall health of your child's hair depends upon many factors, most of them controllable. As a rule of thumb, chemicals and children's hair do not mix. Use gentle children's shampoo and conditioner, and don't overdo it with styling and chemical-based products and styling aids. Shampooing the hair too often, even with a mild shampoo, can result in dry hair, breakage, and spilt ends. A build-up of chemicals from hair products can make the hair look dull and lifeless.

How to Prevent Damaging Hair

Blow-drying for too long or at too high a temperature can also have detrimental effects. Kinky or coarse hair especially needs additional moisturizers to stay soft and manageable. Consider using natural oils (such as olive, argan, or shea oil) rather than more chemical-laden moisturizers.

Hot curling irons can weaken and dry hair. Brushing the hair when it is wet can result in breakage. When the hair is wet, it stretches very easily. Use a large-toothed comb to remove tangles when the hair is wet. Too much brushing can cause breakage, especially if the hair is dry or brittle.

If you child has a hair type that is different from yours, hair care may take much longer than you are used to. You can use this to your advantage by, as shared elsewhere in this text, using this as a time to nurture, love, and be close to your child. There is no point in rushing when you can plan an appropriate amount of time to properly care for your child and his or her beautiful hair.

Artificially stretching the hair can cause breakage and hair loss.

Be sensible when using clips, elastic bands, and other styling aids, and do not overuse or leave in for an inordinate period of time. Artificially stretching the hair can cause breakage and hair loss. As the hair moves, it creates friction at these points of contact with the clips and bands, thus weakening the hair. The constant tugging of hair extensions and braids causes stress at the follicle and can result in hair loss.

Poor nutrition can be a contributing factor to poor hair health. Eating a diet that provides the essential minerals and vitamins that the hair requires is necessary. Foods such as meats, eggs, and nuts are rich in vitamins E, C, B complex, B-6—and the minerals of sulfur, magnesium, and zinc—and are known to be especially beneficial to maintaining and growing healthy hair. Whatever condition your child's hair is in, you can improve it.

Processing (Chemicals, Heat, and Ironing/Flattening/Pressing) Hair

The use of chemicals, heat, and other processes can have a negative effect upon the hair of your child or teen. Your child may desperately want to have her hair colored, relaxed, straightened, or curled, but it is up to you to know the risks and help her make choices for healthy hair.

Coloring, perming, or straightening your child's hair can lead to damage or breakage. Bleaching or coloring the hair can weaken the internal bonds that hold it together, resulting in hair loss and breakage. Too much processing of young hair can deplete its natural oils, minerals, and vitamins necessary for healthy hair. Hold off on such processes, if at all possible, until your child is older.

Natural is... Well, Natural

Although slight cosmetic enhancements including makeup, hairstyling, teeth whitening, and braces to straighten teeth are accepted and frequently used in society, there is a danger that your child may develop self-esteem issues if he or she feels that his or her natural hair, face, teeth, and body aren't acceptable without modification.

Historically, people of various ethnic groups, African Americans included, have been judged for their natural hair or other physical features. Your adopted child may have to deal with judgment and criticism of his or her natural hair from people—at school or elsewhere—who are prejudiced. Unfortunately, such cruelty is a part of life. So it is essential that in the home you avoid creating any negative associations with your child's natural hair or other physical attributes. Parental attitudes affect children's attitudes toward themselves and others.

Parental attitudes affect children's attitudes toward themselves and others.

It is essential to educate your child as early as possible (even as a toddler) about personal boundaries and space. Some people (who may mean well) may inappropriately touch your child's hair or examine their hairstyle (particularly if it is elaborate) without permission. Along with a conversation about body parts, good-touch versus bad-touch, and stranger dangers, you should let your child know that his or her head and hair belong to him or her alone.

It is a conversation you'll probably have several times. You'll want to make it clear that Mommy or Daddy or another caregiver may touch their head or hair or body to protect them or care for them, but that the child has a right to decide if he or she wants other people touching his or her head. Don't think that your child is too young to have this conversation. Children can learn to be respectful and yet politely set their boundaries, as well as to respect the boundaries of others.

You don't want your children to grow up disrespecting the boundaries—physical or otherwise—of others, or to feel that someone else can dominate them in any way, whether by touching their hair without permission or otherwise being disrespectful to his or her person. You can make time for these kinds of discussions with your child when you are performing his or her hair-care or skin-care regimen.

In the next section, you'll get guidance in creating a hair-care kit for your child or teen. Remember that this can be a really fun, loving experience and a great way to bond with your child.

Hair-Care Kit

ONCE YOUR CHILD HAS HAIR, which he or she may have from birth, you can make a hair-care kit. If your child is old enough, he or she can help you make it. Making a hair-care kit can become a pleasant bonding experience. Let your child make participate as much as possible. If feasible, have your child decorate the box or bag to give him or her a sense of pride and ownership.

Your hair-care kit should include:

- Wide-tooth or other comb(s)
- Rattail comb (great for parting hair)
- Boar bristle (or other) brush
- Plastic spray bottle (for water)
- Hair clips and/or hair pins
- Leave-in conditioner, hair oil, or other moisturizer
- Scalp moisturizer
- Cloth-coated rubber bands (various sizes)
- Hair ornaments/Hats/Bandannas/Scarves/Sleep caps

After making the hair-care kit, sit down and work with your child's hair. Make this time a positive experience. While you comb and brush your child's hair, be sure to compliment him or her and express how much you enjoy doing his or her hair.

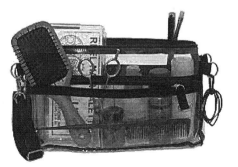

Hair Issues from A to Z

IT IS IMPORTANT TO MONITOR your baby's, child's, or teen's scalp and hair. We all want to be healthy, which includes having a healthy scalp and hair. Additionally, hygiene and physical appearance can affect our self-esteem.

Our physical person is the first thing that people see when we meet them in person. Although judging another based on appearance alone is superficial, it is nevertheless true that people are image-conscious. Again, you may have access to the medical history of your child's biological family, but then again, you may not. Your child may have hereditary issues or sensitivities that could affect the health of his or her scalp and hair. Carefully observing your child's scalp and hair and noting any changes may alert you to a condition (serious or not) that requires treatment.

Generally hair and scalp conditions aren't life-threatening, although they may have truly irritating or concerning symptoms.

Most hair and scalp problems or issues will improve relatively quickly by eliminating contributing factors and treating symptoms. Hair issues are not that common in infants, young children, or teens, but they do occur. Generally hair and scalp conditions aren't life-threatening, although they may have truly irritating or concerning symptoms. Most hair and scalp problems are visible to other people, and so they may affect your child's self-esteem. Some hair and scalp conditions can be more serious, take longer to resolve, or are a sign of a serious medical condition. Hair loss, or alopecia, can be a sign of thyroid disease, an autoimmune disease like lupus or diabetes, a protein deficiency, or even cancer (if it is unrelated to chemotherapy or other cancer treatments).

Use this book if you suspect your child has a hair or scalp condition, and consult your dermatologist if you have concerns that aren't addressed.

Cradle Cap—Seborrheic Dermatitis

AS MENTIONED IN THE SKIN-CARE SECTION of this book, cradle cap is a form of seborrheic dermatitis that is common in babies. Cradle cap affects babies (generally three months of age or younger) and may spread to the skin or folds and creases of the body. Affected skin areas may include the face (including eyelids and eyebrows), chest, belly button, underarms, breasts, and groin area.

Cradle Cap Symptoms

- Mildly reddened, inflamed skin

- Oily/greasy, sometimes weepy or crusty, scalp skin

- Scaly dandruff-like skin flakes (yellow or white) that fall from the scalp

Cradle Cap Causes

Cradle cap may have hormonal causes as well as be the result of overactive oil (sebaceous) glands, whose greasy nature keeps old skin cells, which are naturally shedding or flaking, from falling away normally.

Cradle Cap Treatment

It isn't contagious and can't be cured, but often cradle cap improves with:

- Gentle application of baby oil to baby's scalp, which can soften and loosen scaly bits of skin and then be brushed away with a soft brush.

- Frequent use of a gentle seborrhea shampoo on your infant over six months of age (but be careful to avoid getting it in their eyes).

Avoidance of breaking your child's skin. For example, be especially careful when washing your infant's hair or brushing skin flakes from his skin or scalp. Broken skin is more easily infected.)

PATIENT STORY

I usually see cradle cap in first-time moms who are afraid of the fontanelle (soft spot) on the newborn's scalp. While you don't want to scrub vigorously, I do recommend using a baby's brush to loosen the crust and jojoba oil for the flaking of the scalp.

WHEN TO SEE A DERMATOLOGIST

Have a dermatologist examine your child and recommend treatment if cradle cap recurs or won't go away with over-the-counter solutions (or if it spreads from the head to the face or body). With no cure, frequent shampooing with a gentle product may be your best option.

Dandruff—Seborrhea

DANDRUFF IS AN INFLAMMATORY SKIN CONDITION and a form of eczema called seborrhea. The scalp gets greasy (from natural oils) and has scaly areas (alopecic patches). There's no redness with dandruff, which causes white or yellow flaking of scalp onto the head and hair. Yeast or fungus may build up on the scaly surface of seborrhea-inflamed scalp areas and exacerbate the condition. The condition may spread to the skin around the eyelashes and eyebrows.

Dandruff Symptoms

SYMPTOMS

- Scaly or crusty patches of scalp skin

- Oily/greasy, sometimes weepy, scalp skin

- Dandruff or skin flakes (yellow or white) that fall from the scalp

- Cracked, sometimes itching, scalp skin

- Flaking of skin near eyelashes and eyebrows

Dandruff Causes

CAUSES

One cause of dandruff, as with seborrheic dermatitis, is overactive oil (sebaceous) glands that keep old skin cells, which would naturally shed or flake, from falling away normally. Other causes include having a weakened immune system (from treatment for an illness, such as chemotherapy, or an illness itself), stress, genetic predisposition, or hormonal issues. Overgrowth of *Mallassezia* (a fungus) may cause dandruff and skin inflammation.

TREATMENT

Dandruff Treatment

- Dandruff is not contagious or curable but can be treated. Symptoms often improve with the following treatments (over-the-counter and prescription): Cortisone-based creams and lotions to reduce inflammation

- Medicated over-the-counter shampoos

- Prescription creams to help reduce fungus overgrowth

- Prescription-strength shampoos to help soothe skin

WHEN TO SEE A DERMATOLOGIST

Have a dermatologist evaluate dandruff if it won't go away with over-the-counter solutions or if it spreads from the head to the face or body. Be gentle when cleansing your child's eyelashes, if the seborrhea has spread to this area; soap, shampoo, or prescription medications can seriously harm the eyes. Your teen may be especially concerned about dandruff as some people mistakenly believe dandruff reveals poor personal hygiene. Untreated, dandruff can lead to situations that cause embarrassment. Dandruff may make children susceptible to related bacterial or fungal infections.

Tinea Capitis/Ringworm

TINEA CAPITIS, OR RINGWORM OF THE SCALP, is a fungal infection of the scalp skin. Scalp ringworm develops most often in prepubescent children. Ringworm of the scalp is highly contagious (shared belongings, such as hairbrushes, hats, school naptime cots, and pillows, may be infected); your child must be treated. The scalp may show hair loss or show scaling. Signs of ringworm may appear elsewhere on the body. In other cases, scalp ringworm will present as a large lesion that turns into a rash. The condition may be mistaken for seborrheic dermatitis or eczema.

Tinea Capitis/Ringworm Symptoms

SYMPTOMS

- Inflamed, scaly, hairless patches on the head.
- Hair loss or bald spots (or areas on the head that appear bald).
- Lesions (open and/or fluid-filled) on the face, trunk, or extremities.
- Kerions (round, scaly, tumor-like, boggy skin lesions).
- Itching and/or crusting of the scalp.
- Low-grade fever.
- Swollen neck lymph nodes.
- Brittle hair that breaks off at the surface of scalp.
- A black dot pattern on the scalp (from broken-off hair).

Tinea Capitis/Ringworm Causes

CAUSES

A fungus (one of several types of dermatophytes) living on dead skin cells, or keratin, causes scalp ringworm. A playmate, shared hats or helmets, or contaminated hair-styling tools may spread the disease. "Dandruff" that is not controlled by the treatments suggested above should be evaluated for tinea. Often a scraping (KOH) examination or fungal culture is necessary for proper diagnosis.

TREATMENT

Tinea Capitis/Ringworm Treatment

Your child's dermatologist may prescribe an oral antifungal medication. Sometimes your dermatologist will prescribe Nizoral shampoo (with ketoconazole, an antifungal, as an ingredient) to treat this infection. Ringworm of the scalp must be treated in order to resolve. Because the fungus is down in the hair shaft, treatment generally lasts a minimum of thirty days.

WHEN TO SEE A DERMATOLOGIST

Have a dermatologist evaluate your child and prescribe treatment as soon as you suspect ringworm of the scalp. It won't go away by itself, is highly contagious, and may be difficult to differentiate from other skin conditions. There are different prescription drug treatments, some of which may be taken by mouth.

Folliculitis

FOLLICULITIS IS AN INFLAMMATORY REACTION in one or more hair follicles. In children it is common on the face, the backs of the legs, or the scalp. Bacteria, such as a species of staph (*Staphylococcus*), can then infect the follicles.

Folliculitis Symptoms

SYMPTOMS

- Rash, redness
- Itching, pain
- Pus-filled pustules or pimples (at the hair follicle)
- Oozing of fluid/pus

Folliculitis Causes

CAUSES

Folliculitis is usually caused by some kind of ongoing friction (sometimes from too-tight clothing), an ingrown hair, irritation, an injury such as a scrape, or as a result of an ongoing skin condition such as eczema or dermatitis.

Folliculitis Treatment

TREATMENT

In most cases, folliculitis heals when you:

- Eliminate any infection with prescribed topical antibiotics.
- Avoid the friction that may have caused the issue.
- Avoid too-tight clothing, rubbing, or scratching.
- Avoid using contaminated washcloths.

WHEN TO SEE A DERMATOLOGIST

Have a dermatologist evaluate your child's condition and recommend treatment if you suspect or know your child has folliculitis. It is essential to prevent a folliculitis infection from spreading. Folliculitis responds well to treatment but, as hair follicles are deep, may take some time to heal or may come back and/or spread to other parts of the body. Any contributing or causative bacterial infection, including staph, could be quite serious and must be treated along with the folliculitis.

Head Lice/Pediculosis

A HEAD LOUSE IS A PARASITE that is found on the head. Different from body lice, head lice (plural of louse) infestation is common among children and is very contagious. Anyone who comes into contact with an infected person or their contaminated belongings, including clothing, hair brushes, combs, or bedding, is at risk of being infected. Head lice will not go away without treatment, but there is no reason to panic if your child is infected (or reinfected). Sometimes an announcement from a child's daycare, school, or summer camp is the first notice a parent has that their child could have head lice. A child can be infested with head lice even if his or her hair is washed regularly and that child has great hygiene. Lice have a preference for straight hair, but it is not unheard of for kinky or curly hair to be affected as well.

Head Lice Symptoms

SYMPTOMS

- Itchy scalp skin
- Crawling scalp sensation
- Sores or red bumps from scratching (less common)
- Tiny nits or lice visible in or on the head and hair

Head Lice Cause

CAUSES

A head lice infection is caused when an adult or juvenile head louse (a nymph), is living on your child's head and feeding on their scalp, and when one or more nits (lice eggs, usually yellow or white and oval in shape, which hatch in about six to ten days after being laid) are present. Nymphs become eggs seven days or so after hatching and live by feeding on your child's blood, which can cause itching in some children.

PATIENT STORY: *LICE, OH MY!*

Once your children start school, they often bring little "gifts" home to the family. I had a family come in with their two adopted young children, one caucasian (6) and the other African American (4)—both were in school. Mom brought the children in to discuss treatment for lice, as there had been an outbreak at school with the dreaded note sent home. We talked about the condition and treatment, and I advised the mom to treat everyone in the family, including the adults in the home.

I shared with her my own experience with the dreaded note from school, going undercover into our local pharmacy to purchase the lice kit, hiding the kit under other items in my cart and praying there was not a price check at the register and that I would not run into patients or friends that day! The kit is easy to use, but I suggested she might use different techniques based on the hair types (wider tooth comb for the curly hair). Interestingly, lice are less common in curlier hair, presumably because the oils used on curly hair and the oil on the scalp of curly hair is a less hospitable environment for lice to survive and thrive. Adding some rosemary oil to the scalp may also deter re-infestation.

TREATMENT

Head Lice Treatment

Getting rid of head lice can be difficult. A louse can survive up to three days (off a human body). You will have to treat your entire home and everyone living in it, which means cleaning all furniture, toys/stuffed animals, bedding/rugs, clothing, body care products (combs/brushes), car seats. You can vacuum to remove all adult lice, nymphs and eggs, and loose infected hairs from the carpet, rugs, floor, and furniture. Shake off and bag up items (in plastic) that can't be washed and dried. Bedding towels and clothing will need to be washed in hot water. Combs and brushes can be soaked in hot water for at least fifteen minutes. You will also need to treat your infected child and family members.

Eliminating lice can be daunting. It takes a lot of effort to completely get rid of an infestation. There are no shortcuts. Your child will only get reinfected if you fail to eliminate a head lice infestation from your environment (both your home and automobiles). Remove your child from a childcare situation that is infested with lice until that environment is clean, or they will just get reinfested.

In most cases, head lice are treated by/with:

- Removal of head lice (adults, nymphs and eggs) by hand.

- Over-the-counter lice shampoo (for children *OVER* the age of two).

- A special fine-toothed comb designed for lice nit removal.

- Treatment of all belongings including bedding/towels.

- Avoiding sharing hair accessories or grooming tools with others.

- Use of prescription lice treatments (in severe cases that don't resolve).

WHEN TO SEE A DERMATOLOGIST

See a dermatologist if your child has lice and is a toddler or infant. Also, dermatologists can diagnosis an asymptomatic child (a youngster without obvious symptoms). So see your doctor if you think your child might be infested with lice (perhaps you received a note from a child care provider or school mentioning an outbreak of lice). Your doctor may prescribe an antibiotic if your child has developed a bacterial infection or has a rash or scabs from scratching. Do not use products for lice that haven't been medically approved. There are prescription lice treatments which may be available if over-the-counter products are not effective, but they do come with US Food and Drug Administration consumer warnings and shouldn't be used on children who are too young. Do not use over-the-counter lice medication, including shampoos, without physician guidance if you are pregnant or your child is a newborn or younger than three years of age.

Hair Loss

HAIR LOSS OR THINNING NATURALLY OCCURS AS PEOPLE AGE and may be hereditary, but genetic hair loss is generally seen in older adults and not in babies, children, or teens. Typical hair loss can be around fifty to one hundred hairs daily and can vary seasonally. Just like all animals, we tend to "shed" more in the spring and fall. Babies often lose the hair they have at birth, generally called "baby hair," sometime during the first six months of life. Infants may develop bald spots or even lose most or all of their hair. However, it does grow back.

Your child may have thinning, breaking, damaged, or slow-growing hair for a number of reasons. Hair loss may result from improper styling techniques or inadequate nutrition, which can be easily resolved. However, loss of hair may result from disease or a serious underlying condition. Seek medical treatment if your child is experiencing hair loss. Hair loss in children can occur slowly, over a period of months or weeks, or quite rapidly.

Hair Loss Symptoms

SYMPTOMS

- Hair loss (excessive)
- Bald patches on head
- Gradual thinning of hair

Hair Loss Causes

CAUSES

Alopecia Areata—
A condition in which loss of hair, generally in patches, occurs due to an autoimmune disorder when hair follicles are attacked and damaged by a person's own immune system.

Chemotherapy—
Given to a child as part of a cancer treatment plan; can cause the side effect of hair loss.

Iron Deficiency Anemia—
Can cause hair loss or increase the normal shedding of hair and can occur if your child has been lacking in specific vital vitamins and minerals. Certain children adopted internationally may be susceptible to iron deficiency anemia (as well as malnutrition and/or rickets).

Medication—
Many medications can cause hair loss.

Improper Nutrition/Malnutrition

Telogen Effluvium—
Loss of hair due to an interrupted, abnormal hair growth cycle so that most or all hairs are thrown into the telogen hair-growth phase–and baldness, or partial baldness, results. This type of hair loss can occur quite rapidly, over a few days, in response to a stressful event, which precedes the hair loss by about ninety days.

Thyroid Disease—
Whether overactive or underactive, can cause hair loss.

Tinea Capitis—
Or ringworm of the scalp, sometimes causes hair loss.

Traction Alopecia—
Is a hair loss issue due to hair-line or hair-shaft trauma from overly tight hairstyles (frequent/constant wearing of too-tight braids, ponytails, or other styles) or frequent/constant processing of the hair.

Trichotillomania—
A scalp and hair condition resulting from loss of hair due to obsessive pulling, rubbing, or twisting (individuals with this condition often pull out hair from their scalp, eyebrows, and eyelashes). This form of hair loss often requires treatment by a mental health professional to identify underlying source of stress precipitating this obsessive-compulsive behavior.

TREATMENT

Hair Loss Treatment

Treatment for hair loss includes:

- Identification of reason for hair loss.

- Treatment of emotional or other issues leading to hair twisting/pulling.

- Adequate nutrition (if vitamin/nutrient deficiency is an issue).

- Use of laser brush or comb (or other device) to stimulate hair growth.

- Steroid treatment (if loss is caused by alopecia areata inflammation).

WHEN TO SEE A DERMATOLOGIST

If you can't easily identify and avoid the cause of your child's hair loss, you should consult with a dermatologist. You must know the cause of your child's hair issue in order to treat it effectively. In some cases, hair loss may not require treatment, although treatment may stimulate hair regrowth. A dermatologist can diagnose reasons for hair loss, offer treatment options, and explain what outcomes to expect.

Hair Damage

HAIR DAMAGE IS CAUSED BY hair products and practices that are too harsh for that particular head of hair. This may include over-washing, use of too much heat when blow-drying or using flat irons, or over-processing with chemicals. If your teen is damaging or destroying his or her hair with the use of particular tools or products, encourage him or her to stop using the destructive items. After healthy new hair grows, he or she can be careful to avoid damaging it. The ingredients in chemical relaxers (with or without lye) and other products such as permanents, dyes, and straighteners can be extremely damaging to the hair follicles and hair itself.

Your child's ethnic background may mean that his hair is more likely to break or be damaged by the use of certain products (or the failure to use certain products such as moisturizers). Avoid styling techniques that are inappropriate for your child's hair type. Hair may require both protective styling and protection while sleeping. A breathable fitted cap or scarf, ideally made from silk or satin, can minimize or prevent hair loss or breakage. Cotton sheets absorb natural hair oils and dry out the hair.

Hair Damage Symptoms

- Hair loss or thinning
- Breaking or splitting
- Extremely dry, rough, or brittle texture
- Dullness (little shine)

Hair Damage Causes

Situations or things that may cause hair and/or scalp problems include:

- Illness
- Emotional stress, depression, or anxiety
- Poor nutrition leading to vitamin or other nutritional deficiency
- Overuse of heat styling tools
- Tightly pulled hairstyles
- Breakage from friction or rubbing

SYMPTOMS

CAUSES

- A burn or other injury
- Hair pulling or twisting (trichotillomania)
- Medical treatment (such as chemotherapy, radiation, or surgery)
- Exposure to chemicals (permanents, dyes, straighteners, relaxers)

Hair Damage Treatment

TREATMENT

- Reduce or eliminate emotional stress, depression, or anxiety.
- Treat emotional or other issues leading to hair twisting/pulling.
- Get adequate nutrition (if vitamin/nutrient deficiency is an issue).
- Determine allergies, if any, contributing to hair loss.
- Avoid use of damaging hair tools.
- Allow time for hair regrowth (after medical treatments, etc.).
- Use appropriately gentle hair products (no harsh chemicals).

WHEN TO SEE A DERMATOLOGIST

Unless you can easily identify and avoid the cause of your infant's or child's hair damage, you should consult with a dermatologist. Knowing the cause of your child's hair issue will allow you to treat it effectively.

Scalp Damage

SCALP PROBLEMS, WHICH ARE GENERALLY NOT SERIOUS, may be caused by any number of things. The ingredients in chemical relaxers, permanents, dyes, and straighteners can be extremely damaging to the hair and scalp. Certain shampoos and conditioners may contain harsh ingredients that can strip the protective coating of chemically treated hair and harm the hair or scalp.

Scalp Damage Symptoms

- Extremely itchy scalp skin.
- Chafing or red scalp skin.
- Fever or pain in combination with scalp issues.
- Bumpy texture or blisters and sores on scalp.
- Red streaks from a spot or sore on scalp.
- Bleeding or pus draining from scalp.
- Loss of clumps or patches of hair.
- Odor.
- Scalp build-up different from natural skin tone.

Scalp Damage Causes

- Illness.
- Emotional stress.
- Poor nutrition leading to nutritional deficiency.
- Heat styling tools (straightening, curling, drying, or other tools).
- A burn or other injury.
- Hair pulling or twisting.
- Medical treatment (such as chemotherapy, radiation, or surgery).
- Chemicals (permanents, dyes, hair straighteners, relaxers).

Scalp Damage Treatment

At-home treatments for scalp damage can be helpful and are recommended. The following treatments can be helpful to eliminate scalp issues.

- Eliminate the use of harsh chemicals.

- Reduce or eliminate emotional stress.

- Treat emotional or other issues leading to hair twisting/pulling.

- Treatment for fungal or other scalp infections.

- Adequate nutrition (if vitamin/nutrient deficiency is an issue).

- Avoid damaging hair tool use.

- Allow for time to heal from medical treatments.

- Use medicated shampoos.

WHEN TO SEE A DERMATOLOGIST

Unless you can easily identify and avoid the cause of your child's scalp issues, you should consult with a dermatologist. Scalp damage may be caused by illness, so it's important to pay attention to your child's hair and scalp and seek medical attention for the symptoms of scalp damage.

<u>Conclusion</u>

THE LOVE AND CARE YOU GIVE your adopted children provides them a foundation of self-esteem based in self-acceptance and self-love, all because you are teaching them to care for their skin, hair, bodies, and beings. Have fun with your child but seek treatment immediately if you suspect he or she has a skin, scalp, hair, or other medical issue or condition.

Skin Resources

aad.org

The American Academy of Dermatology, founded in 1938, is the largest dermatologic association in the world, with more than 16,000 dermatologist members. Their website offers expert skin care and condition information, including articles, research, and online videos, as well as free skin-care programs (like free skin cancer screenings and a no-cost summer camp for kids with skin disease).

sundicator.net

The Sundicator is a simple-to-use online UV calculator that allows you to choose the UV index value (a scale from 1-11 that represents risk level of skin damage due to UV exposure), your skin phototype, the SPF of the sunscreen you will use, your location, and the weather. With a click of the mouse, you will find out how long you can safely stay in the sun after proper initial application of your sunscreen.

sunaware.org

SunAWARE has multiple projects, one of which is the production and distribution of children's books that teach about skin cancer prevention and detection. The group distributes the books for free to schools and programs that do not have the budget to buy them. Visit their website for free articles and other resources on being safe in the sun.

SUNPRECAUTIONS.COM

COOLIBAR.COM

SUN PROTECTIVE CLOTHING

sunprecautions.com

Solumbra's fabric provides 30+ SPF all-day sun protection and many of the garments made of Solumbra are designed with special pockets and mesh panels, so that warm air exhausts and cool air is allowed in. Solumbra is a four-way stretch fabric that provides 30+ UVA and UVB sun protection, blocking more than 97 percent of UVA and UVB rays. Solumbra is considered a medical device (intended for the prevention of disease).

coolibar.com

Fabric with a UPF of 50 allows only 1/50th of the UV radiation falling on the surface of the garment to pass through. This means it blocks 98 percent of UV radiation. All Coolibar brand garments rate UPF 50+, the highest possible rating. Coolibar is another company that makes sun protective clothing. Their products offer 50+ UPF (ultraviolet protection factor), and they have clothing for men, women, children, and infants from six months of age.

SKIN CARE PRODUCTS

- **aveeno.com**
- **cerave.com**
- **cetaphil.com**
- **eucerinus.com**
- **sebamedusa.com**
- **pisco.com/vanicream**

LAUNDRY DETERGENTS FOR SENSITIVE SKIN/SKIN ISSUES

- **all-laundry.com**
- **cheer.com**
- **dreft.com**

Hair Resources

ONLINE RESOURCES FOR HAIR PRODUCTS, STYLING SUGGESTIONS

THE INTERNET CAN BE A FANTASTIC RESOURCE for adoptive parents, particularly in the area of hair care and hairstyling. If you are a parent who has adopted a child with a different genetic background, skin tone, and hair texture, then you may want to read articles and watch videos online about how to style or care for your child's particular type of hair. There are many great resources. Some of my favorites are:

- **chocolatehairvanillacare.com**
- **curls.com**
- **kinky_curly.com**
- **naturallycurly.com**

Skin & Hair Glossary

ALLERGY

An **allergy** is a body sensitivity and response to a substance, food, or ingredient, and may result in swelling, sneezing, inflammation, or other immune system reactions.

ALOPECIA

Alopecia is hair loss from the body or head.

APOCRINE GLAND

An **apocrine gland** is a sweat gland and is usually near, or associated with, a hair follicle.

ESTHETICIAN

An **esthetician** is a professional who is trained and skilled in treating facial skin with beauty products and in giving beauty treatments such as facials.

SKIN ERUPTION

A **skin eruption** is a "breaking out," such as with a rash, red spots, or other skin symptom.

FACIAL SKIN

Facial skin is the skin on your face. A spa treatment for the face is often referred to as "a facial."

HAIR FOLLICLE

A **hair follicle** is a part of the scalp or skin out of which one or more hairs grow.

IMMUNE SYSTEM

The **immune system** is a part of the human body that helps protect the body by causing particular responses, under certain circumstances, in response to certain pathogenic organisms or substances that the body recognizes as harmful.

INFECTION

Infection occurs when pathogenic organisms, such as bacteria, viruses, or fungi, contaminate body tissue, migrating and growing.

INFLAMMATION

Inflammation is swelling of body tissue often accompanied by redness. It may be hot and/or painful.

PRURITIS

Pruritis is an itch, a feeling that makes one want to scratch the skin.

SCALP

The **scalp** is the skin on the head that has hair follicles from which hair, generally, grows outward.

STEROID

A **steroid** is an anti-inflammatory and anti-itch medication used in a variety of skin disorders.

WOUND

A skin **wound** is an abrasion, laceration, cut, scrape, puncture, tear, or other break in the skin's surface. Accidents, violence, disease, or surgery may wound the skin.

<u>Appendix</u>

FIGURE 1: THE SKIN AND HAIR

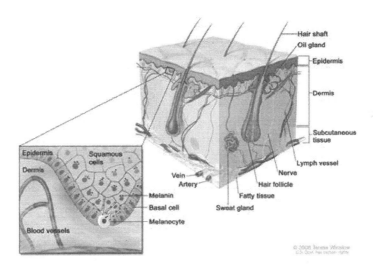

Index

A

Aboriginal peoples, skin color, 1–2

accessories, hair, 78–79

acid, hair conditioners, 67

acne

    facial cleansing, 13

    facials, 7

    neonatal and infant, 26–29

    overview of, 30–31

adolescents. *See* teenagers

African Americans

    hair care, 33

    melanoma, 51

    natural hair, 81

    skin color, 1–2

allergies

    defined, 107

    sunscreen, 50

alopecia areata, 68, 96–98, 107

American Academy of Dermatology (AAD), 104

anxiety

    acne and, 30–31

    eczema, 19

    scalp damage, 101–102

apocrine gland, 107

arsenic, 58

Asians

    hair care, 33

    melanoma, 51

atopic dermatitis, 18–21, 50

Australians, skin color, 1–2

B

bacterial infection, 25, 34

baldness, 69

barrettes, 78

basal cell skin cancer, 56–59

bathing, 6, 7, 20. *See also* shampoo

Bi-racial children, hair care, 33

birthmarks

    café au lait spots, 45–46

    vascular birthmarks, 41–44

blisters, sunburn, 54

braids, hair care, 76

Brazilians, skin color, 1–2

brushes, hair, 65

bubble baths, 6–7

C

café au lait spots, 45–46

cancer, skin

    moles, 35–36

    pediatric skin cancer, 56–59

    sun damage, overview, 51–52

    sunscreen use, 8

canthardin, 38

Caribbean peoples, skin color, 1–2

Caucasian children, hair care, 33

chemicals, hair care, 80, 101–102

chemotherapy, 96–98

children

    hair loss, 68

    ringworm, 88–89

    skin care basics, 9–13

    sunburn, treatment for, 53–54

    sunscreen, 8

cleansers

    acne and, 13

    eczema, 20

    shampoos, 65–66

    skin, 5–6

    skin-care kit, 14

    use of, 11

clips, hair accessories, 78

color, hair, 80

color, skin, 1–2

combs, 65

conditioners, hair, 67, 72

contact dermatitis, 50

cradle cap, 32–33, 84–85

cryotherapy, 37

curling irons, 79–80

curly hair, 74–75

D

dandruff, 32–33, 86–87

dermatopathologist, 57

diaper rash, 24–25

diet, hair and, 61, 80, 97

discoloration

    acne and, 31

    birth marks, vascular, 41–44

    café au lait spots, 45–46

dry shampoo, 66

dry skin, 5–7, 16–17. *See also* eczema

E

eczema, 18–21, 86–87

electrosurgery, 37

esthetician, 107

Index (continued)

F

facials, 7

flat irons, 80

folliculitis, 90–91

fragrances, in products, 20

fungal infection

    dandruff, seborrhea, 86–87

    diaper rash, 25

    overview, 34

    tinea capitis, ringworm, 88–89

G

genetic disorders, neurofibromatosis, 45, 47–48

H

hair

    accessories for, 78–79

    basic care tips, 70–72

    braids, simple, 76

    cradle cap, seborrheic dermatitis, 32–33, 84–85

    curly, kinky, wavy, care and styling, 74–75

    dandruff, seborrhea, 86–87

    folliculitis, 90–91

    frequently asked questions, 64–69

    hair damage, 99–100

    hair loss, 96–98

    hair-care kit, 82

    head lice, pediculosis, 92–95

    natural hair, 81

    overview, 61, 83

    preventing damage to, 79–80

    processing, 80

    puffs, 77

    resources, 106

    scalp damage, 101–102

    straight hair, care and styling, 73

    tinea capitis, ringworm, 88–89

    twists, care of, 75–76

    types of, 62–63

    washing recommendations, 33

hair follicle, defined, 107

hairbrushes, 65

head lice, 92–95

head wraps, 79

headbands, 79

hemangioma, 41–44

Hispanics, hair care, 33

human papilloma virus (HPV), 37–38

I

immune system

    defined, 107

    eczema, 19

    warts, 38

Indians, skin color, 1–2

infants

    acne, 26–29

    birth marks, 41–44

    cleansers, 5–6

    cradle cap, 32–33, 84–85

    diaper rash, 24–25

    hair, 62

    hair loss, 68, 71

    moisturizers, 5–7

    skin care basics, 9–13

    sunburn, treatment for, 53–54

    sunscreen, 8, 50

infections

    defined, 108

    diaper rash, 25

    folliculitis, 90–91

    molluscum contagiosum, 39–40

    overview of, 34

    warts, 37–38

inflammation, defined, 108

intertrigo, 24–25

iron deficiency, 97

itching

    diaper rash, 24–25

    eczema, 18–21

    head lice, 92–95

    keratosis pilaris, 22–23

J

jaw clip, 78

K

keratin, 61

keratosis pilaris (KP), 22–23

ketoconazole, 89

kinky hair, 74–75

L

laundry detergent, 20

lice, 92–95

M

Malassezia furfur, 32, 86–87

melanocytes, 1–2

melanocytic nevi (moles), 35–36, 41–44

Index (continued)

melanoma
  pediatric skin cancer, 56–59
  sun damage, overview, 51–52
Middle Eastern descent, skin color, 1–2
moisturizers
  hair, 67
  skin, 5–7, 14
moles, 35–36, 41–44
molluscum contagiosum, 39–40

N

natural hair, 74
neonates. *See also* infants
  acne, 26–29
  birth marks, 41–44
  cradle cap, 84–85
  hair, 62
  hair loss, 71
neurofibromatosis, 45, 47–48
Nevus flammeus, 41–44
newborns. *See* neonates
Nizoral shampoo, 89
Northern Europeans, skin color, 1–2
nutrition, hair and, 61, 80, 97

P

PABA (para-aminobenzoic acid), 50
pediatric skin cancer, 56–59
pediculosis, 92–95
photoallergic dermatitis, 50
phototypes, 3–4
port-wine stain, 41–44
poxvirus, 39–40
pruitis, 108
puffs, hair care, 77

R

rashes, 7, 24–25
ringworm, 88–89

S

scalp, damage to, 101–102. *See also* hair
scarring, acne, 31
scarves, 79
sebaceous glands
  acne, 30–31
  seborrheic dermatitis (dandruff), 32–33, 86–87
seborrhea, 86–87
seborrheic dermatitis, 32–33, 84–85
self-esteem, building
  birth marks, treatment for, 44
  hair, 62
  overview, 4
shampoo
  double-stranded twists, 75–76
  overview, 65–66, 72
  seborrheic dermatitis (dandruff), 33
Shea butter, 6–7
skin
  care basics, 9–13
  color, 1–2
  cradle cap, seborrheic dermatitis, 84–85
  healing and, 1
  moles, 35–36
  resources, 104–105
  skin-care kit, 14
  skin-care products, 5–8
  types (phototypes), 3–4

skin cancer
  moles, 35–36
  pediatric skin cancer, 56–59
  sun damage, overview, 51–52
  sunscreen use, 8
skin eruption, defined, 107
snap clip, 78
soap. *See* cleansers; shampoo
SPF, sun damage overview, 49–52
squamous cell skin cancer, 56–59
steroids
  defined, 108
  long-term effects, 32
  seborrheic dermatitis, 32
straight hair, 73
strawberry mark, 41–44
stress
  acne and, 30–31
  eczema, 19
  scalp damage, 101–102
sun protective clothing, 105
SunAWARE, 104
sunburn and suntan
  information resources, 104–105
  skin types, 3–4
  sun damage, overview, 49–52
  sun protection kit, 8, 55
  symptoms and treatment for, 53–54
Sunindicator, 104
sunscreen
  application of, 8, 11
  infants, 9
  skin-care kit, 14
  sun damage, overview, 49–52
  sun protection kit, 55

Index (continued)

T

tanning. *See* sunburn and suntan

teenagers

    acne, 13, 30–31

    facials, 7

    skin care basics, 9–13

    sun damage, overview, 50–52

telogen effluvium, 68, 97

texture, hair, 62

thyroid disease, 97

tinea capitis, 88–89

traction alopecia, 97

trichotillomania, 68, 97

tweens

    acne, 13, 30–31

    facials, 7

    sun damage, overview, 50–52

twists, hair care, 75–76

U

UV rays. *See also* sunscreen

    pediatric skin cancer, 57

    sun damage, overview, 49–52

    sun protection kit, 8, 55

    sunburn, symptoms and treatment, 53–54

    Sunindicator, 104

V

vascular birthmark, 41–44

viral infection

    diaper rash, 25

    molluscum contagiosum, 39–40

    overview, 34

    warts, 37–38

von Recklinghausen disease, 47–48

W

warts, 37–38

wavy hair, 74–75

wet shampoo, 66

wound, defined, 108

X

xerosis cutis, 16–17

Y

yeast, 32

young children

    cleansers, 5–6

    moisturizers, 5–7

About the Author

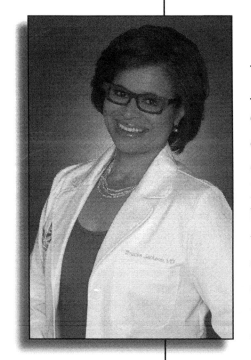

DR. BROOKE JACKSON

BROOKE JACKSON, M.D., born and raised in Washington, DC, is a graduate of Wellesley College and Georgetown University Medical School. Upon completion of her pediatric internship at University of Chicago and dermatology residency training at Henry Ford Hospital, Dr. Jackson was the first African American dermatologist to be awarded laser fellowship training at Harvard University, where her interests and research helped to pioneer the uses of lasers in ethnic skin. She completed a second fellowship in skin cancer surgery (Mohs micrographic surgery) at Baylor College of Medicine in Houston, Texas, then joined the staff of the MD Anderson Cancer Center, where she founded the Mohs Surgery Unit and served as its director until relocating to Chicago. She founded the Skin Wellness Center of Chicago, where she serves as the medical director, and holds a clinical appointment in the department of dermatology at Northwestern University Medical School.

A board-certified dermatologist and dermatological surgeon, Dr. Jackson is a member of the American Academy of Dermatology; the American College of Mohs Micrographic Surgery and Cutaneous Oncology; and the American Society of Dermatologic Surgery. She is the author of numerous articles, book chapters, and a CD-ROM relevant to her specialty. A laser surgery expert, she lectures nationally on the use of lasers and cosmetic procedures in ethnic skin. Dr. Jackson's other clinical interests and expertise includes the prevention and treatment of skin cancer, and cosmetic procedures. She formerly served as national treasurer of the National Medical Association Dermatology section.

A gifted communicator, Dr Jackson is a frequent contributor to local and national media. She has appeared on ABC, CBS, NBC, Fox, and WGN news, and has been quoted frequently in print media, including *O The Oprah Magazine, Essence, Glamour, Self, Shape, Fitness, Parents,* HuffingtonPost.com, and mommymdguides.com. She also writes a recurring column for *Heart and Soul* magazine.

An avid runner and budding triathlete, she has completed ten marathons and eight triathlons. In 2010, she was selected to represent the

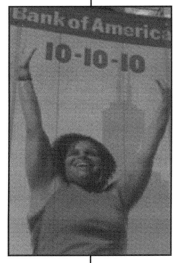

Bank of America Chicago Marathon for 10-10-10 as part of their campaign celebrating ten runners who give back to their community. (*On the right is a portion of an ad for the 2010 marathon that graces a building at North Avenue and I-94 in Chicago.*) In 2000, she organized and directed Chicago Fit, a marathon training group of four hundred that met in Hyde Park until 2004. She is a board member of Girls on the Run, a national organization that helps girls ages eight to eleven to build self-esteem through sports. Dr. Jackson currently serves as a Pre-K class mother for her son and a Daisy troupe leader for her girls.

LEARN MORE ABOUT DR. JACKSON AT
www.brookejacksonmd.com

Acknowledgments

I wish to thank my parents, Aeolian and Marvin Jackson,
who taught me how to be a compassionate human being;

Dr. Edward Krull, my mentor and friend,
who showed me how to be a compassionate physician;

and the birth mothers of our children,
who have given me something amazing:
the opportunity to be a compassionate and loving mom.

~Brooke Jackson, M.D.

20486005R00067